Zebra

An Aid to Obscure Diagnosis

By the author:

In Print:

Zebra Cards: An Aid to Obscure Diagnosis

The Astronaut Almanac: Volumes 1 and 2

The Physical Lincoln

The Physical Lincoln Sourcebook

On the Web:

`www.doctorzebra.com`

`www.expertmapper.com`

`www.physical-lincoln.com`

Zebra Cards™

An Aid to Obscure Diagnosis

John G. Sotos, MD

Mt. Vernon Book Systems
Mt. Vernon, Virginia
1991+

This is a 2006 reissue of the 1991 printing of *Zebra Cards*. To simplify production, simple page-printing is used instead of perforated card stock, and the two volumes are combined into one. Nothing else from 1991 is altered, except that the introductory material is paginated differently and includes a few minor textual changes, explained by footnotes. Occasional "special editions" with different covers contain the same contents.

The author is grateful to the American College of Physicians, the original publisher, for taking a chance on *Zebra Cards*. It has been a pleasure working with them over the years. The author is also grateful to the ACP for returning copyright, so *Zebra Cards* can once again be made available.

Visit us at:
`www.zebracards.com`
`www.mtvernonbooksystems.com`

Third printing, 2006, with minor changes
Second printing, 1991, with revisions
First printing, 1989

Printed in the United States of America

The cards and introductory material were produced using the TEXtures and TEXShop implementations of the TEX typesetting system. TEX is a trademark of the American Mathematical Society. TEXtures is a trademark of Blue Sky Research. TEXShop is by Richard Koch and Dirk Olmes, and includes work by Gerben Wierda.

Library of Congress Control Number: 2008933537
ISBN 978-0-9818193-0-3 (third printing)

Table of Contents

To my Mother and Father

Introduction

When you hear hoofbeats behind you, don't expect to see a zebra.

– Dr. Theodore E. Woodward *(1)**

Despite its absence from medicine's formal lexicon, the term **zebra** is used in the medical community both commonly and with near-universal comprehension *(2)*. On the rare occasions when it does appear in print, understanding of its meaning is usually assumed or is given by reprinting an analogue of the canonical quotation above *(3)*. Thus, lacking a formal definition for the term, I will try to provide one here.

Zebra is frequently equated with a rare disease or condition. This conceptualization is too restricted, however. Consider the following events, reported by a physician who took his daughter to the 1978 Worcester, Massachusetts science fair and carnival *(4)*:

> We heard a sudden sound of hoofbeats, followed by screams from the crowd. Expecting horses, I was *surprised* to see that two small zebras, pulling a cart, had gotten away from their handlers and were running amok.

The italics are added to emphasize surprise as the essence of the experience. "Surprise" is defined as: 1. an unexpected encounter, or 2. a feeling of astonishment or amazement *(5)*. This leads directly to our definition for **zebra**: A medical condition whose appearance at a particular time and place, in a particular person, is both unexpected and astonishing. The "condition" may be an item from the history, a physical finding, a laboratory result, or a diagnosis. Casual reflection reveals that rare diseases do, in general, satisfy this definition *(6)*; slightly more thought shows that

---

* The 1989 and 1991 printings attributed this saying to "Anonymous." I spoke with Dr. Woodward in 1995. Then emeritus chief of medicine at the University of Maryland, Dr. Woodward disclosed that the original late-1940s saying had been "Don't look for zebras on Greene Street," that being the street on which the University of Maryland Hospital was (and is) located.

commoner afflictions may also qualify, if they present in an unusual fashion (for example, card HE-004).

With a more detailed consideration of zebras left for later in the Introduction, let us shift focus to the educational benefits of *Zebra Cards*: What can they teach us, and why is that material important?

I. *Zebra Cards* serve as a motivating force.

Enjoyment of a subject stimulates intellectual exploration and growth. Flipping through the Cards immediately discloses that they are *fun*; this is inherent in the notion of astonishment underlying them. Given the important role that motivation plays in the challenging, occasionally tedious task of learning medicine, it is my hope that the mental stimulation and enjoyment derived from the cards (and the Extracts) will become transformed into an eagerness to study mainstream medicine independently using more conventional sources.

II. *Zebra Cards* teach medical facts.

This is the *raison d'être* for most medical textbooks and, ultimately, for *Zebra Cards* as well. But because the facts presented in *Zebra Cards* are likely to be ignored or glossed over (or even mis-stated) in many textbooks, some colleagues have labeled these cards as a medical equivalent of "Trivial Pursuit." Make no mistake, triviality is a comparative term, applied appropriately to populations and inappropriately to individuals. As McKusick *(7)* has noted in commenting about rare diseases, "It is no consolation to the victim of the disorder that he is one in a million. He still has a right to as thoughtful management as the patient with a run-of-the-mine condition."

III. *Zebra Cards* will sharpen clinical skills.

By example and by repetition, *Zebra Cards* attempt to modify subtly the way a physician thinks during the interview and examination of a patient; that is, to make him or her aware that *anything* could be a clue to the identity of the patient's malady. The same sentiment was well expressed by the English neurosurgeon Wilfred Trotter *(8)*:

> We come ... to the question of what aspects of human faculty it is necessary for the good doctor to cultivate. ... The first to be named must always be the power of attention, of giving one's whole mind to the patient without the interposition of oneself. It sounds simple, but only the very greatest of doctors ever fully attain it. It is an active process and not either mere resigned listening or even politely waiting until you can interrupt. Disease often tells its secrets in a casual parenthesis.

Zebra Cards help attune the physician's ear to the casual parenthesis by showing how the most inconsequential, outrageous, innocuous, or inconsistent statement or observation may be a manifestation of disease. It is well known that a common cause of incorrect diagnoses is failure to consider the proper diagnosis *(9)*. The flash-card format forces the reader to repeatedly think at the boundaries of his or her knowledge. Thus, after a few passes through *Zebra Cards*, the habit of continously asking oneself "What am I missing?" or "What haven't I considered?" will develop. In this way the physician automatically begins using *all* the available data in decision making, and, with this questioning attitude, takes nothing for granted.

That there is a need for reinforcing this manner of thinking is clear: The accelerating pace of activities demanded by the practice of medicine today is the natural enemy of the casual parenthesis. I suspect most (if not all) physicians, of whatever age, are haunted by a feeling that one's professional forebears were somehow vastly more adept than he or she at interpreting the signals of disease *(10)*. Certainly, bemoaning a perceived contemporary decline in clinical skills is not a new practice. For example, Dressler *(11)*, in a 1960 article about the value of percussion in detecting pericardial effusions, quotes the 1936 lament of Sir John Parkinson: "No longer shall we tell of the professor who by knocking at the front door could find out who was in the drawing room."

IV. *Zebra Cards* convey the boundless subtlety of the human organism.

Because common things occur commonly, it is easy in any type of medical practice to fall into an unthinking routine. Osler warned against this brand of hubris *(12)*:

> We, the doctors, are so fallible, ever beset with the common and fatal fallacy of reaching conclusions from superficial observations and constantly misled by the ease with which our minds fall into the ruts of one or two experiences.

Zebra Cards convincingly show, not only at an intellectual level, but at a visceral level as well, that there are subtleties in even the most mundane situations and that no two experiences are ever identical. This knowledge results directly in better patient care and a more enriched practice of medicine *(13)*.

V. *Zebra Cards* help train the mind to remember disjoint facts.

Unlike some of the physical sciences, where a basic set of laws captures a large proportion of the knowledge about a field, medicine lacks grand unifying principles *(14)*. As a result, physicians are required to memorize thousands of facts, too many of which are little used and exist in isolation, with no contextual associations to assist recall. For example, either you know that shoulder pain may be referred from the diaphragm or you do not. Extended work with *Zebra Cards*, I have found, helps develop a facility for remembering unconnected facts that is useful in both medicine and other endeavors.

Zebra Cards should be enjoyable to physicians and students at all levels of clinical experience. They were compiled from an urban North

American internist's point of view. Pediatric conditions are omitted unless the internist has occasion to encounter them. Although neurology's heritage lies in internal medicine, it has developed into a field so arcane and highly refined that it seems as if *everything* in that domain is a zebra *(15)*. I have, therefore, deliberately restricted the number of neurologic cards.

For those readers eager to plunge into the cards, I suggest first reading the following two sections of the introduction; they contain valuable information about the use and misuse of the cards. Beyond the next two sections lies material of potential interest to those who develop a deeper interest in our subject, or who have a philosophical bent.

Happy hunting.

How to Use the Cards

It is simple to use *Zebra Cards*. The front of each card (also called the obverse) lists an observation that one could make in clinical practice, that is, an item from the history, a physical finding, a laboratory result, or a diagnosis. After reading and digesting this item, the reader should construct a differential diagnosis in his or her mind, then inspect the reverse side of the card where the "true" differential appears in italics. Explanatory remarks immediately follow the differential list.

For those wishing to completely understand the format and content of *Zebra Cards*, all seven data fields of a card are briefly described here:

System (obverse, upper left corner) – The cards are filed alphabetically according to system and, in some cases, subsystem (for example, "Mouth-Tongue" is system Mouth and subsystem Tongue.) When the observation presented spans two or more systems, the more "important" system (sometimes an arbitrary choice) is used *(16)*; the index will be of use when problems of partial recall arise. Note that the noun form of the organ is usually used as the system name, not the adjective ("heart" not "cardiac"), and that sometimes there are "parallel" systems ("abdomen" and "GI"). The systems were organized using the headings from the standard review of systems as a model. The choice of subsystems was driven by convenience.

Index number (obverse, upper right corner) – Each card has a unique index number, composed of the first two letters (usually) of its system name, followed by three digits (for example, MO-801). If there is a subsystem, it determines the first of these digits. The last two digits are merely counters. The index, which endeavors to be complete, refers to cards by these index numbers.

Observation (obverse, center) – This is the presenting complaint, item from the history, physical finding, or laboratory result. Although trying to specify the differential diagnosis of the observation necessarily resembles the "What am I thinking?" game that is so unpopular among students and teachers, it does have the advantage of stimulating thought. In many cases you may think of something quite reasonable that is not mentioned in the differential. In this case, I urge you to write me, being sure to provide references. Remember, the idea is to think *before* turning the card.

Eponym (reverse, top center, in parentheses) – Most cards do not have associated eponyms. When they do, the eponym refers to the observation, not to the item(s) on the differential. In some cases the entry in the eponym field is not an eponym, but a medical word whose meaning corresponds to the observation (*eg*, "aniridia" corresponds to the observation "no iris").

Differential (reverse, italicized) – The purpose of *some* cards is to present an exhaustive differential (for example, in cases where the observation elicits in most minds only one or two possibilities, as with card NE-002: delayed relaxation of deep tendon reflexes). With other cards, a complete differential is impossible to give, owing to its length, and a single (surprising) item is selected for discussion (as in card TH-202, gynecomastia). I have tried to limit the number of cards in this class and, in less obvious instances, have included a comment stating that the true differential is much larger. In most cards, however, the exhaustive differential has never been compiled in the literature, and would be extremely laborious to research. In these instances, I present a partial differential (which contains the major items), and solicit help from readers.

Comments (reverse, center) – This will usually be an explanation of the link between the observation and the differential, perhaps followed by a discussion of "related" topics. In some cases the zebras are so hard to believe that all I can do is carefully reprint what the references say (for example, the Searls sign, card NC-002).

References (reverse, bottom) – Extraordinary care has gone into documenting the source of each zebra. A fair number of the items mentioned in the cards are part of medicine's oral tradition. These "facts," unquestioningly passed from one generation of houseofficers to another, can all too easily become distorted over time. I hope that increased accessability to written material will reduce unintentional spreading of misinformation. (For example, I was taught that delayed relaxation of deep tendon reflexes is pathognomonic of hypothyroidism, but see card NE-002). In a few instances the source was not verifiable, but the zebra was so appealing it was included anyway. These cases are explicitly noted. Areas of speculation are clearly indicated. Most footnotes are annotated, and may occasionally contain interesting information apart from their reference. I have made an effort to cite references that are generally available in medical libraries, but this is not always possible *(17)*.

Besides providing a vehicle to encourage thinking, three by five cards have other advantages over conventional textbooks. First, they are easily expanded by the reader. Second, their small size ensures that only key concepts are presented and helps minimize mental fatigue. Third, their size also makes it convenient to take the one or two cards relevant to a particular case, place them in a shirt pocket, and go to the library to scrutinize the references.

As mentioned in the next section, zebras are intrinsically easy to remember. But how can these seemingly unrelated pieces of information be merged into one's corpus of medical knowledge? One useful technique is to pick out a few cards a week and explore these zebras with your patients that week. Thus, for one week you will look for a blue line on the gums of all patients (card MO-704), even if they are complaining of knee pain. You will see no blue lines, of course, but you will gradually appreciate the spectrum of normality in gums, and be ready to recognize a blue line when one finally does present itself. With many of these cards it is impossible to judge something as abnormal unless a prior effort has been made to delineate for oneself what "normal" is (Harvey's fourth precept).

Perhaps the most profitable way to use *Zebra Cards*, however, is as the nucleus for your own expanding collection of cards. The physical format of the cards makes this trivial, while their intellectual format makes it a project that can be sustained (with benefit) for years. In addition, I welcome suggested additions to *Zebra Cards* (see the section called "An Invitation").

In summary, *Zebra Cards* achieves its desired effect on the reader's thinking by three mechanisms:

1. Keeping the reader off-balance. It is one thing to passively read about a disease entity and its complications, but quite another to attempt working through problems (however small) oneself.

2. Demonstrating the richly varied failure modes of the human body. All of us have seen patients with complaints so odd that we dismiss them as functional, thinking "I never heard of anything that will do that." Although I do not agree with the belief that "if the patient says it, then it must be presumed to be true" *(18)*, I think the student of *Zebra Cards* will become (properly) uncomfortable about dismissing complaints as functional in the future.

3. Reinforcing the primacy of the history and physical examination *(19)*. Study of the details mentioned in these cards will, I hope, lead to increased attention to detail in all phases of clinical work, and with it, a renewed confidence in the data gained without benefit of the laboratory.

How Not to Use the Cards

If you cannot think of at least three ways to abuse a tool, then you do not understand how to use it.

– the Count to Three Principle *(20)*

Cognitive psychologists have recently identified some basic mental processes, called heuristics, that humans seem to use as rules of thumb when reasoning on the basis of uncertain data. These mental strategies work well most of the time, but they are not perfect. The *availability heuristic* is of direct relevance to us *(21)*: "Events more easily remembered are judged more probable." Two thousand years ago a similar heuristic was discovered: "The striking and novel stay longer in the mind" (see the Extracts).

These two heuristics are synergistic, and could spell trouble for Zebra Card readers in early stages of their medical training. Zebras are, by definition, striking and novel, and therefore easy to remember; thus, they will tend to appear in differential diagnoses with excessive certainty. One must always be very wary of this. It is essential that zebras appear on the differential when appropriate, but it is *more essential* that the more likely diagnoses all appear on the differential as well. The only way to ensure you can construct such differentials is to give first priority to studying mainstream medicine ("the horses").

Thus, to read *Zebra Cards* without studying the corresponding general sections in textbooks is a potentially damaging misuse of the cards. Osler *(22)* once wrote: "To study the phenomena of disease without books is to sail an uncharted sea." Going to sea with *Zebra Cards* alone is akin to having a chart showing only a few small, widely spaced portions of a long journey's route *(23)*.

When reading the cards, keep two important facts in mind: First, these are not conventional flashcards; if, on your first pass through the cards you try to guess the "answer" to each card, you are bound to be frustrated. Second, do not try to read the cards cover to cover in one sitting; the cards are designed to be approached in small bits at a time. Ideally, the situation will be like the experience we have all had of looking up a word in a dictionary, only to first encounter a different word whose exotic appearance compels us to look it up immediately, which then prompts us to look up yet a different word, and so forth.

Attention to detail is important in medicine, and, to some extent, *Zebra Cards* revel in detail. The cliché says it all, however: "Don't lose the forest for the trees." Immersion in a mass of details can be dangerous. The "big picture" (another cliché – but a useful one) must always be the focus toward which the bulk of energy and thought are directed; for Zebra Cards to suggest otherwise would be a travesty. When a critically ill patient with idiopathic hypertrophic subaortic stenosis becomes your responsibility, do not devote long loving minutes to seeking and/or discussing the Brockenbrough sign – managing the patient comes first.

Finally, important caveats must be directed toward objectivity and honesty, the loss of which can be manifest in ways both insidious and catastrophic. Metaphorical examples of the former include: (i) hearing hoofbeats and *hoping* to see a zebra; (ii) seeing a horse, refusing to acknowledge it, and claiming there could still be a zebra out there; and (iii) seeing something you are pretty sure is a horse, but calling it an "atypical zebra." You will hear hoofbeats often, but see zebras infrequently. This should diminish neither the enjoyment of learning about them, nor the appreciation of horses. If we saw zebras too often, they would cease to be unexpected.

Zebras and Related Equines *(24)*

The world's most widely known physician is probably not William Osler, but Sir Arthur Conan Doyle, the Scottish general practitioner who penned the tales of Sherlock Holmes at the turn of the century *(25)*. I had long been dimly aware that the famous detective's fantastic observational and deductive skills were drawn from a medical model *(26)* (see also the Extracts), but when, as a first-year medical student at Johns Hopkins, I heard upperclassmen relate amazing stories of the diagnostic acumen of Tumulty and the encyclopedic knowledge of McKusick, Holmes' feats suddenly did not seem so stratospheric after all *(27)*.

With this frame of mind, the specific impetus that launched *Zebra Cards* occurred the next year, during the introductory course in clinical skills. I still remember clearly the feeling I had when I first learned of the standard review of systems question, "How many pillows do you sleep with?" The idea that physicians could somehow assess cardiac function by using pillows was, in my mind, fantastic. That I was now privy to this secret, and would soon be let in on others like it, was exhilarating. It was then I began collecting "elegant" clinical signs, which soon coalesced into the concept of zebras.

The succeeding years have made it clear that zebras are not static: They vary as one's knowledge accumulates. No one but a second-year medical student would think of the association between heart failure and orthopnea as a zebra. A third-year medical student thinks the association of gingival hypertrophy with phenytoin use is a zebra, while the third-year medical resident does not. Zebras also change as medicine changes. In a 1928 address, Archibald Garrod *(28)* had hoped "to have spoken of that malady involving the bone-marrow, of which the copious excretion of Bence Jones protein is a diagnostic sign, for it is one of the most obscure of rare diseases." Today, "obscure" is not a word that describes multiple myeloma. Syphilis, the great imitator of a generation ago, is now relegated to zebra in most differential diagnoses; immunodeficiency is not.

We have been careful to distinguish zebras from mere rare diseases, but a brief foray into the literature of rare diseases is instructive, as the field is closely allied with our own. As the Extracts show, some of the brightest stars in the history of medicine have had a special interest in rare diseases, including Hutchinson, Harvey, Paget, and Garrod. Books specifically adressing rare diseases and lesions have appeared *(29-34)*, and others are so enriched with uncommon entities that they serve as invaluable resources, as their frequent citation in these cards attests *(35-38)*. Most of these works devote at least some space to justifying the study of rare diseases, a practice that continues even today, in the era of the omnivorous biomedical research establishment *(39)*.

The points made in these justifications tend to fall into one of a few general arguments. McKusick *(7)*, in his Foreword to Bean's 1967 *Rare Diseases and Lesions*, enumerates them. He lists four reasons (one of which was alluded to previously) "that rare conditions are, or should be of interest to physicians":

- Rare disorders can teach us much about the normal or about more common disorders.
- Rare manifestations are sometimes valuable clues to the existence of grave internal disease.
- People have them.
- They are a break in the routine and "keep [the physician's] powers of observation from undergoing atrophy."

It is simple to see that these justifications may be applied equally well to zebras; for the proof of the first three arguments, one need only look in the cards (*eg*, HE-004 for the first argument, and GI-001 for the second).

Though it has long been known that the rarity of a disease actually makes it rarer *(40)*, and recently stated why "classic cases" are rare *(41)*, there is a mathematical question regarding rare diseases that I have not seen discussed. The devoted student of rare conditions, F. Parkes Weber *(42)*, noted that "For one common disease or syndrome there are several rare ones." Might it then be true that, lumping these rare disorders into a single entity, it is a common occurrence for someone to be suffering from a rare disease *(43)*?

Points of Style

To include all this material in one volume it has been necessary to throw some of it into smaller type.

– Fielding H. Garrison *(44)*

The physical format of *Zebra Cards* is a constant temptation to commit barbarisms against the English language by trying to fit just one more thought into the limited space available for text. Despite implacable resolve, the more important goal of unambiguity may have caused me to yield to such temptations on occasion. Readers are welcome to identify transgressions of grammar or exposition. The cards and the manual were prepared as camera-ready copy, using the TEXtures implementation of Donald Knuth's TEX typesetting system on an Apple Macintosh. The addition of illustrations, while obviously desirable, would have ensured the work's noncompletion; seek out the references.

It seems that in every compendium of dissimilar medical facts, the author(s) take a stand regarding the use of eponyms. With some trepidation, I admit that I am *for* them. In many cases, a name is easier to grasp than a string of medicalese words. Attention to eponyms can teach much about the history of medicine (including the notion of unfairness, which many eponyms are). Eponyms have the additional advantage of not attaching pathophysiologic labels to poorly understood phenomena prematurely; this is especially desirable when operating at the fringes of knowledge, as we do here *(45)*. I do agree, however, that, except in a few cases too deeply entrenched to be changed, the posessive form of the eponym should be avoided *(46)*.

[The Fat Man] was the only resident to have his own reference file on every disease there was, on three-by-five cards. He loved references on three-by-five cards. He loved everything that was on a three-by-five card.

– *The House of God (47)*

An Invitation

The present revision of this book has been made as exhaustive and searching as has been possible in the extra-official time at the author's disposal.

– Fielding H. Garrison *(48)*

An individual can no longer expect to master all knowledge in internal medicine during a normal lifespan *(49)*. This is especially true when operating at the level of detail found within these cards. A central tenet of computer science, however, holds that switching from serial processing of information to parallel processing can substantially improve task performance. Thus, I invite all readers to become parallel co-processors of data, and submit their favorite zebras for possible inclusion in the next edition of *Zebra Cards*. The address is: `hoofbeats2006@zebras.com`*

After eagerly poring through *Zebra Cards* countless times, readers will, I hope, gain an appreciation of what makes a good card (and what does

* *Zebra Cards* was the first medical book to include an email address for soliciting comments. In 1989 email spam did not exist. To evade the spammers, the numerical part of the `hoofbeats2006` address will be incremented each year.

not). To minimize the amount of frustration and nonproductive effort, however, some general principles are listed below:

1. A rare disease does not a Zebra Card make; we seek little known, but striking manifestations of any disorder, be it rare or common. Thus, Mollaret meningitis is a rare condition, but it has no symptom or sign sufficiently striking to set it off from other chronic meningitides. The manifestation must be reasonably obscure; every medical student knows that "sterile pyuria" occurs in renal tuberculosis, even though renal tuberculosis is nowadays rare.

2. Manifestations with long differentials should, in general, be avoided. Thus, nephrotic syndrome after an insect sting is unsuitable because listing "nephrotic syndrome" as the observation calls an extremely long differential to mind. This can sometimes be circumvented by mentioning a specific population in the zebra, for example, "nephrotic syndrome in a neophyte beekeeper" (ugh!). When many of the items in the differential have occurred only at the case report level of frequency, an approach similar to card EA-006 (calcified pinna) may be adopted.

3. It is *imperative* that each zebra be referenced as completely as possible.

4. No pediatrics, please (all those congenital syndromes!), unless untreated or undiagnosed patients have been reported to live past adolescence. As previously mentioned, neurology is a zebra-rich environment, so submissions in this category will be judged more stringently.

Even if you do not have a zebra to submit, any form of nonviolent communication will be eagerly accepted, including suggestions and criticism, both specific and vague.

Finally: It was stated at the Outset, that this system would not be here, and at once perfected. You cannot but plainly see that I have kept my word. But I now leave my [classification] System standing thus unfinished, even as the great Cathedral of Cologne was left, with the crane still standing upon the top of the uncompleted tower. For small erections may be finished by their first architects; grand ones, true ones, ever leave the copestone to posterity. God keep me from ever completing anything. This whole book is a draught nay, but the draught of a draught. Oh Time, Strength, Cash, and Patience!

Herman Melville [1851]
– *Moby-Dick (50)*

Acknowledgments

At a tender age, four or five years give a man a local attachment to place and teachers which is very natural, very nice, but not always the best thing for him. He goes out with a strong bias already in his mind, and is ready to cry, "I am of Guy's," "I am of Bart.'s," or "I am an Edinburgh man." To escape from these local trammels, which may badly handicap a man by giving him an arrogant sense of superiority often most manifest when there is least warrant, is very difficult.

– Osler *(51)*

Many before have felt inadequate in trying to express the profound debt owed their teachers; I must now add my name to that list. Despite Sir William's words above, I am not hesitant to admit that this work is very much a product of the unique environment of the Johns Hopkins Hospital Department of Medicine *(52)*. Foremost among its contemporary architects are Dr. Victor A. McKusick and Dr. Philip A. Tumulty, whose Olympian accomplishments and personal qualities continue to foster the Hopkins traditions of caring and clinical excellence. Only in the supportive, stimulating environment created by these two men could *Zebra Cards* have reached fruition. It is a lucky person indeed who has the opportunity to work with his personal heroes.

Other members of the faculty have been greatly influential, in particular Drs. John Michael, Stephen Achuff, Kenneth Baughman, and H. Franklin Herlong. Dr. Thomas Traill's current job description is inadequate; to reflect his true activities, another item must be added: routinely astonishing fellows, houseofficers, and students with the amount of information extracted from the physical examination. I will never be able to sufficiently thank Nick Belitsos for all he has done for me; I will pay for the door, however.

Unfortunately, I must content myself with naming only a few of the residents on the Osler medical service from 1980 to 1984 who taught me so much as a student and intern. Rick Munschauer, Bruce Gelman, and Jerry Granato showed me early on what a good Marine was supposed to be. Hugh Rienhoff's encouragement was greatly appreciated. Mike Schindler and Bill Balke were incredibly patient during that incredible August on incredible O3. Rick Lange, Kevin Fox, and Alison Freifeld always took an interest in the cards. The finest qualities of the physician, embodied in the Assistant Chiefs of Service, are typified by Peter Holt, Susan MacDonald, Steven Schulman, and Hacib Aoun, to each of whom I owe so much.

My debt to the other 37 members of the 1983-84 Osler intern group is incalculable and unforgettable.

The agile mind of John Leonard was the source of numerous ideas. Peter Belitsos, Rich Embrey, Dave Borislow, and John Brofman tolerated my occasional (?) ramblings with amazing good humor. Steve Holland, Gina Dallabetta, Mindy Shapiro, and Ray Wilson engaged in helpful discussions, and my brother George has become a valued contributor and critic as he progresses in his medical training. To the members of the Pithotomy Club and the RACC: You probably delayed the completion of this project by a year or two, but I would not have had it any other way. The zebra-seeking zeal of Marc Litt is appreciated. To the physicians, pararescue section, and others in the 129 ARRG, CA-ANG who so broadened my outlook on medicine (and the world), all I can say is: Move east.

I am grateful to Drs. Thomas Traill, Stuart Selonick, and Frederick Bustin for reading the manuscript and greatly improving *Zebra Cards* with their ideas. The responsiblity for errors, however, is mine alone. Thanks also to the staffs of the Welch Medical Library at Hopkins and the Lane Medical Library at Stanford for providing outstanding research resources, and especially to Professor Peter Travis of Dartmouth College, who, too long ago, taught me how to write a paragraph.

The greatest teachers of all, however, are my parents. Their unflagging wisdom, love, and encouragement are the foundation, not only for this project, but for everything I have attempted. Thank you, Mom, and Thank you, Dad ... for everything.

Abbreviations

The abbreviations below may be encountered in the text without an accompanying explanation:

AS	aortic stenosis
ATP	adenosine triphosphate
CDC	Centers for Disease Control
CNS	central nervous system
CPC	clinico-pathological conference
CSF	cerebrospinal fluid
EKG	electrocardiogram
GI	gastrointestinal
GU	genitourinary
Ig	immunoglobulin
LV	left ventricle
MI	myocardial infarction
PAT	paroxysmal atrial tachycardia
PVC	premature ventricular contraction
RV	right ventricle
TB	tuberculosis
UCSF	University of California, San Francisco
WPW	Wolff-Parkinson-White syndrome

Extracts

(with apologies to Herman Melville)

To be hurt is part of the game.

– *The Healing Hand (53)*
[page 1]

As a rule, lightning diagnoses are to be disparaged; often dramatic, they may prove dangerous.

– Hamilton Bailey *(54)*

Now when the neighboring doctors found
    A case so rare had been descried,
They every day her ribs did pound
    In squads of twenty; so she died.

– The Stethoscope Song *(55)*
Oliver Wendell Holmes

It's obvious or it's not there.

– Leonard's Law of Physical Findings *(56)*

What one knows, one sees.

– Goethe *(57)*

"Dr. Knight became interested in physical diagnosis when he realized the grave errors physicians were making in determining the size of the gastric gas bubble. As a result of his great concern, he spent a year at one of the country's leading abdominal gas clinics, where he had an opportunity to master this intricate skill. By golly, when Dr. Knight percusses a gastric bubble, you can believe his results! He reports it to the millimeter! He is one of the few people working on the diurnal variation of gastric bubble size."

"What happens if the patient burps?" asked Alice.

"Dr. Knight becomes very angry!" said Dr. Lizard, starting to quake at the thought. "He makes a terrible scene – hours of labor down the drain! However, the patients are usually cooperative, because they fast before the gastric percussion and cannot eat during the procedure, which takes several hours."

– from "Up the Bronchial Tree" *(58)*

Newly discovered knowledge, even if it is trivial to some, is rarely trivial to the one who discovers it.

– Robert Petersdorf *(59)*

Where we see in every day life things that are pretty, ordinary, and banal, we generally fail to remember them, because the mind is not being stirred by anything novel or marvelous. But if we see or hear something exceptionally base, dishonorable, unusual, great, unbelievable, or ridiculous, that we are likely to remember for a long time.... Ordinary things easily slip from the memory while the striking and the novel stay longer in the mind.

– from *Ad Herrenium (60)*
[ca. 85 BC]

Try to learn the features of a disease or injury, gentlemen, as precisely as you know the features, the gait, the tricks of manner of your most intimate friend.

– Joseph Bell, MD *(61)*
[1837-1911]

Joseph Bell, MD, FRCS ... was 39 years old when [Arthur Conan] Doyle entered Edinburgh University in 1876 to read for the degree of Bachelor of Medicine.... Doyle became Bell's "out-patient clerk," which meant that in the waiting room he made simple notes of each case before showing the patients, one by one, into the big room where Bell sat in state, surrounded by his dressers and students.

"He would sit in his receiving room," wrote Doyle, "with a face like a Red Indian, and diagnose the people as they came in, before they even opened their mouths. He would tell them their symptoms, and even give them details of their past life; and hardly ever would he make a mistake."

The results were often dramatic, as in the following dialogue between Bell and a civilian patient, recorded by Doyle in his autobiography:

'Well, my man, you've served in the army.'

'Aye, sir.'

'Not long discharged?'

'No, sir.'

'A Highland regiment?'

'Aye, sir.'

'A non-com. officer?'

'Ayc, sir.'

'Stationed at Barbados?'

'Aye, sir.'

'You see, gentlemen,' he would explain, 'the man was a respectful man, but did not remove his hat. They do not in the army, but he would have learned civilian ways had he been long discharged. He has an air of authority and is obviously Scottish. As to Barbados, his complaint is elephantiasis, which is West Indian and not British.'

[In another case,] a woman with a small child was shown in. Joe Bell said good morning to her and she said good morning in reply.

'What sort of crossing di'ye have fra' Burntisland?' [said Bell in "rich Scots."]

'It was guid.'

'And had ye a guid walk up Inverleith Row?'

'Yes.'

'And what did ye do with th' other wain?'

'I left him with my sister in Leith.'

'And would ye still be working at the linoleum factory?'

'Yes, I am.'

'You see, gentlemen, when she said good morning to me I noticed her Fife accent, and, as you know, the nearest town in Fife is Burntisland. You noticed the red clay on the edges of the soles of her shoes, and the only such clay within twenty miles of Edinburgh is in the Botanical Gardens. Inverleigh Row borders the gardens and is her nearest way here from Leith. You observed that the coat she carried over her arm is too big for the child who is with her, and therefore she set out from home with two children. Finally, she has a dermatitis on the fingers of her right hand which is peculiar to the workers in the linoleum factory at Burntisland.'

[In] one of the best of these stories, ... Bell observed that a patient "had the whole appearance of a man in one of the Highland regiments." The patient, a shoemaker, retorted that he had never been in the army in his life, a denial which Bell conceded "was rather a floorer." When the patient stripped, however, a small blue "D" branded on his skin was discovered under his left breast. He had been a deserter from the Crimean war, a fact which pride had naturally caused him to wish to conceal.

– from "The Origin of
Sherlock Holmes" *(62)*

A CAT scan was performed to confirm that Presidential Press Secretary James Brady had been struck in the head by a bullet.

– CBS News reporter covering
the Reagan assassination
attempt *(63)*

"You see that?" asked Dr. Lizard, pointing to a dark-green pouch stuffed into one of Dr. Knight's pockets.

"Yes," said Alice.

"Well, that is a chemical kit for finding bile in the sputum," said Dr. Lizard. "It is an invention of his own!"

"Bile in the sputum?" repeated Alice.

"Yes, of course!" declared Dr. Lizard. "Dr. Knight believes that all body secretions should be fully examined and, therefore, one of the special research interests in this hospital is bile in the bronchial tree. Why, we are almost at the point of finally discovering that rare and most important cause of biliptysis."

"What is that?" asked Alice.

"Ectopic gall bladder, of course!" exclaimed [Dr. Lizard] as if Alice had just demonstrated a severe supratentorial synaptic deficiency.

"Why everyone knows that the lungs and the gall bladder are both diverticula from the gut tube! Therefore, it is easy to see that there could be a congenital anomaly where the gall bladder got mixed up and grew off too high, ending up in the lungs by mistake.... In gall bladder ectopia a very experienced clinician would percuss a local area of dullness which varied with the fat content of the previous meal (Knight's sign). An occasional patient might appear with a history of violent wheezing and coughing fits to which some ignorant physician had no doubt affixed the diagnosis of 'atypical asthma' which, on careful review of the data, are clearly intermittent cholelithiptysis, caused by pulmonary cholelithiasis."

"I cannot imagine that your yield of positive sputum tests is high enough to make the test worthwhile," said Alice.

"I suppose you would be willing to let a case of asymptomatic biliptysis go by unnoticed!"

– from "Up the Bronchial Tree" *(58)*

When you don't know what's going on, always save urine.

– Stephen Spielberg, MD *(64)*

Frankly to confess ignorance is often wiser than to beat about the bush with a hypothetical diagnosis.

– Osler *(65)*

Back off, man; I'm a scientist.

– Bill Murray in *Ghostbusters*

The material which an active consultant may collect in a long lifetime is enormous. The late Dr. Austin Flint's notes cover 16,922 folio pages, all written in his own hand.

– Osler *(66)*

[F. Parkes] Weber (1863-1962) remained active at the Royal Society of medicine until after the age of 90 years and he was frequently called upon to resolve difficult diagnostic dilemmas by virtue of his legendary knowledge of rare disorders. It is recorded in his obituary that when, for the first time in his life, he stated at a meeting of the Society that he had "never heard of the syndrome" which was under discussion, tumultuous applause broke out, followed by cheers and stamping of feet; the noise reached a crescendo and the meeting was abandoned in disorder!

– from *The Man Behind the Syndrome (67)*

Nor bring to see me cease to live
    Some doctor full of phrase and frame,
To shake his sapient head, and give
    The ill he cannot cure a name.

– Matthew Arnold *(68)*

How is it that, one fine morning, Duchenne discovered a disease which probably existed in the time of Hippocrates?

– Charcot *(69)*

One picture is worth 1024 words.

– Anonymous

Pluralitas non est ponenda sine necessitae.

– William Ockham *(70)*
[ca. 1280 - 1349]

To know things well, one must know them in detail, and as this is infinite, our knowledge is necessarily superficial.

– LaRouchefoucald *(71)*

Errors in medical reasoning are obviously due to the same cause which the great intellect of Spinoza assigned for all human mishaps: "inadequate ideas."

– Fielding H. Garrison *(72)*

If this is not the correct diagnosis then, as Dr. [William S.] Thayer used to say, it just goes to prove that the best diagnosis is not always the correct diagnosis.

– A. McGehee Harvey *(73)*
(upon making the diagnosis of Hansen disease at a clinicopathologic conference)

There are both within and without the body many other kinds of structures, which differ from one another as to sufferings both in health and disease;

such as whether the head be small or large; the neck slender or thick, long or short; the belly long or round; the chest and ribs broad or narrow; and many others besides, all of which you ought to be acquainted with, and their differences; so that knowing the causes of each, you may make the more accurate observations.

– Hippocrates *(74)*
[ca. 400 BC]

In making the diagnosis of the cause of illness in an individual case, calculations of probability have no meaning. The pertinent question is whether the disease is present or not. Whether it is rare or common does not change the odds in a single patient.... If the diagnosis can be made on the basis of specific criteria, then these criteria are either fulfilled or not fulfilled.

– A. McGehee Harvey,
James Bordley III, and
Jeremiah Barondess *(75)*

Addison's disease may be classed amongst the least rare of rare maladies.

– Archibald Garrod *(28,76)*
[1928]

Nature is nowhere accustomed more openly to display her secret mysteries than in cases where she shows traces of her workings apart from the beaten path; nor is there any better way to advance the proper practice of medicine than to give our minds to the discovery of the usual law of Nature by careful investigation of cases of rarer forms of disease. For it has been found, in almost all things, that what they contain of useful or applicable is hardly perceived unless we are deprived of them, or they become deranged in some way.

– William Harvey *(77)*
[1657]

We are told that in France, at the time of the first empire, when the French universities were in the melting-pot, there were established, in some of the medical schools, professorships for the exposition of rare cases and diseases.... In our own medical journals and transactions I have found only two addresses on the subject [of rare cases], but the authors of these were both giants... Sir James Paget and Sir Jonathan Hutchinson.

– Archibald Garrod *(28)*

Amongst the infinitely varied derangements of structure and function which make up the total of human maladies we have some which are constantly before us, and others are so infrequent that a man may live through a long professional life and scarcely see a single example of them. All will admit that the first must be studied as a matter of duty by every conscientious practitioner, but respecting the latter there is a wide-spread and very natural feeling that it does not matter whether we understand them or not.

It is against this form of apathy that I wish to protest to-night, and I am not without hope of making it clear that these varieties are often the most instructive; that they stand in close relationship to the common, and that it is the duty of all, so far as possible, to understand them, and to try also to further the knowledge of them.

– Sir Jonathan Hutchinson *(77)*
[1889]

But even as they are, singly and in disorder, we ought not to set [rare cases] aside with idle thought or idle words about "curiosities" or "chances." Not one of them is without meaning; not one that might not become the beginning of excellent knowledge, if only we could answer the question – Why is this rare? or, being rare, why did it in this instance occur?

– Sir James Paget *(77)*
[1882]

We may feel sure that, in the future as in the past, there will be many who will try to solve the problems of the commoner diseases, the control of which is of such vital interest to the community at large. Let us hope that there will always be some who will seek to guess the riddles and to learn the lessons of the rarer maladies.

– Archibald Garrod *(28)*

To talk of diseases is a sort of Arabian Nights' entertainment.

– Osler *(78)*

Regard yourselves as indomitable gatherers of clinical evidence. Hunt for it anywhere it might be hidden, in the history or physical examination, in some special test, or in a conversation with a family member, or tucked away in some previous medical report, for hidden anywhere it may well be.

– Tumulty *(79)*

Nowadays, in contrast to the past, a diagnosis must often be specifically correct if the patient is to get well, for so many modern forms of therapy have highly specific actions. This scientific advancement compels the clinician to sharpen his clinical skills to the very keenest edge, so that he can extract from a meticulous history and physical examination every particle of pertinent clinical evidence, which he then co-ordinates with evidence gathered by other means. Never before has such a premium been placed upon expertise in the performance of the history and physical examination as the prime steps in the diagnostic process from which all other investigative steps logically proceed.

– Tumulty *(79)*

In science we are interested in things, not in persons.

– Marie Curie *(80)*

Care more particularly for the individual patient than for the special features of the disease.

– Osler *(81)*

A pair of kidneys will never come to the physician for diagnosis and treatment. They will be contained within an anxious, fearful, wondering person, asking puzzled questions about an obscure future, weighed down by the responsibilities of a loved family, and with a job to be held, and with bills to be paid.

– Tumulty *(82)*

References

We may state that we are following the distinguished model of Pierre Beyle, whose footnotes are four times as extensive as his text

– Hans Zinsser *(83)*

Note: Looking up each footnote while reading through the Introduction is not recommended. They serve only to provide references and as an opportunity to discuss tangents without breaking the flow of the main text.

1. Anonymous to this author, at least. The phrase has been ascribed to Philip Tumulty of Johns Hopkins, but in a May 1982 conversation with me, he denied coining it. It appears to have been extant at least as early as 1960 (PJ Imperato. *Medical Detective*. New York: Richard Marek; 1979:13, 18). Can anyone out there help?

   The adage, "Common things most commonly occur," has been attributed to Samuel Gee (1839-1911); see *Circulation*. 1954;**10**:574-9.

2. The following medical dictionaries were consulted: Stedman's 24th edition, Dorland's 26th, Blakiston's 4th, Urdang's first, Taber's 15th, Black's 32nd, and the *Dictionary of Medical Slang and Related Esoteric Expressions* (JE Schmidt. Springfield, Illinois: Thomas; 1959). The canonical quotation has even been used on NBC-TV's television show "St. Elsewhere."

3. The quotation is briefly discussed in: DM Eddy, CH Clanton. The art of diagnosis. *N Engl J Med*. 1982;**306**:1263-8. Variations are common as well, for example, *Ann Intern Med*. 1986;**105**:138. See also *The House of God* (reference 47), pages 46-7 and 335.

4. WJ Nagel. Striped horses [Letter]. *N Engl J Med*. 1980;**303**:1005.

5. Only slightly altered from P Davies, ed. *The American Heritage Dictionary of the English Language*. New York: Dell; 1969.

6. The distinction between rarity and surprise is detailed in: W Weaver. Probability, rarity, interest, and surprise. *Pediatrics*. 1966;**38**:667-70.

7. Page vii of *Rare Diseases and Lesions* (reference 29).

8. JB Wyngaarden, LH Smith Jr, eds. *Cecil Textbook of Medicine*. 16th ed. Philadelphia: WB Saunders; 1982:xxxiii-xxxiv.

9. See, for example, the study of 100 consecutive autopsy-proven myocardial infarctions in which only 53 were correctly diagnosed antemortem [*JAMA*. 1983;**250**:1177-81.].

10. Someone told me a story about Burrill Crohn (as in Crohn disease) who, as an old man, was hospitalized for some ailment, and during his recuperation was invited to join rounds with the ward team one morning. At the conclusion of rounds, one of the house officers asked him "Dr. Crohn, tell me, what was it like in the days when giants walked the halls?" To which Crohn replied, "I don't know. When I was an intern, my residents told me that those days had already passed."

11. *J Am Med Assn*. 1960;**173**:761-4. This is the Parkinson of Wolff-Parkinson-White, not of Parkinsonism.

12. Teacher and student. In: W Osler. *Aequanimitas With Other Addresses to Medical Students, Nurses and Practitioners of Medicine*. 3rd ed. Philadelphia: Blakiston; 1932:21-41.

13. For an example of this philosophy in action, see Tumulty's introduction to *The Effective Scutboy*. 3rd ed. (RH Harrell, GS Firestein, eds. East Norwalk, Connecticut: Appleton & Lange; 1988).

14. Here, the word "medicine" does not mean "patient care," where, of course, unifying principles do exist. Instead, it refers to the scientific and pathophysiologic knowledge that forms the basis for sound patient care.

15. This is not complete hyperbole. In a *New England Journal of Medicine* clinicopathologic conference where the final diagnosis was metachromatic leukodystrophy, 36 different diseases were mentioned in the case discussion. Of these, I had never even *heard* of 19 (*N Engl J Med*. 1984;**310**:445-55). Others, too, have commented on the "many, diverse disorders of obscure origin that affect the central and peripheral nervous systems" (JB Martin. Whither neurology? *N Engl J Med*. 1984;**311**:-1048-50.).

16. In the case of cutaneous signs, they are entered under system "Skin" only if the location of the sign is of small consequence. Compare cards SK-001 and TH-001.

17. Space considerations dictated the telegraphic format of the cards' citations, which are adapted from McKusick's catalogs of inherited traits (reference 38). When the reference is unlikely to be standard library fare, the citation is amplified. Entries in *Mendelian Inheritance in Man*

are cited by concatenating "McKusick" and the catalog entry number, for example, "McKusick 31206" is properdin deficiency (card IM-005). The multi-volume *Handbook of Clinical Neurology* is cited as if it were a journal. To maximize legibility, neither book nor journal titles are italicized in the cards' citations.

While I have faithfully tried to keep the 700 or so references in *Zebra Cards* up to date, the need has not seemed so compelling in the case of some popular textbooks, because these usually reflect information that can easily be updated by the reader. The frequent citation of McKusick numbers is a means to maintain bibliographic currency. The *Scientific American Medicine* textbook would seem to provide a similar means, but the impermanence of its chapters is a problem.

18. EJ Cassell. *Talking with Patients.* Cambridge, Massachusetts: MIT Press; 1985. Reviewed in *N Engl J Med.* 1986;**315**:200-1.

19. H Schneiderman. *Bedside Diagnosis: An Annotated Bibliography of Recent Literature on Interviewing and Physical Examination.* Philadelphia: American College of Physicians; 1988.

20. Alas, I cannot remember where I encountered this fundamental law of the universe, but it may have been in the *Co-Evolution Quarterly* in the mid to late 1970s. The law's importance is alluded to in the current work's subtly ambiguous subtitle.

21. A Tversky, D Kahneman. Judgement under uncertainty: heuristics and biases. *Science.* 1974;**185**:1124-31. The classic article.

22. This famous quote may be found in any of the following: (i) W Osler. Books and men. *Boston Med Surg J.* 1901;**44**:60-1; (ii) W Osler. *Aequanimitas With Other Addresses to Medical Students, Nurses and Practitioners of Medicine.* 3rd ed. Philadelphia: Blakiston; 1932:209-15; or (iii) CNB Camac, ed. *Counsels and Ideals from the Writings of William Osler.* Birmingham, Alabama: Classics of Medicine Library; 1985:159.

23. But not quite as bad as the sea chart in Lewis Carroll's *The Hunting of the Snark.*

24. At the risk of stretching a metaphor too far, we may call an entity that is orders of magnitude more astonishing than a zebra a *quagga.* The quagga was a member of the genus *Equus*, and therefore a relative of both the horse and the zebra. It had stripes only in the front half of its body. The animal has been extinct since the late 1800s.

Amazingly, however, even extinct animals have their days in the sun. A flurry of stories about quaggas recently appeared when DNA from the hide of a (dead) quagga was successfully cloned. See: (i) Blueprint of a lost animal. *Newsweek.* 18 June 1984:64 (illustrated);

(ii) *Science News*. 1984;**125**:356; or (iii) Telling a quagga by its stripes. *Science News*. 1985;**128**:70.

25. An interesting article titled "Doctors in other walks of life" may be found in: J Walton, et al. *The Oxford Companion to Medicine*. Oxford; 1986;I:318-23. (See also the "Doctors Afield" series published in the *New England Journal of Medicine* in the early to mid 1960s.) Physicians who achieved fame outside the biomedical sciences include Copernicus (1473-1543), Thomas Muffet (d. 1604; he wrote a book on insects and has been immortalized in the nursery rhyme "Little Miss Muffet"), Joseph Guillotin (1738-1814), Jean Paul Marat (1743-1793; stabbed in his bath by Charlotte Corday), Peter Mark Roget (1779-1869; as in the thesaurus), Georges Clemenceau (1841-1929), Sun Yat-Sen (1866-1925), and even Pope John XXI (1215-1277).

    The entry about Thomas Young (1773-1829), however, is clearly the most ego deflating. Among other accomplishments, he explained how visual accomodation is achieved by the lens (for which he was elected to the Royal Society at age 21), established the wave theory of light, discovered the principle of intereference of light, gave his name to the modulus of elasticity ("Young's modulus"), and was the first to decipher the Rosetta Stone.

26. I Wallace. The real Sherlock Holmes. In: *Reader's Digest Treasury for Young Readers*. Reader's Digest Association: Pleasantville, New York; 1963:74-6. See also FT Fitzgerald, LM Tierney Jr. The bedside Sherlock Holmes. *West J Med*. 1982;**137**:169-75.

    Sherlock Holmes, by the way, is said to be one of the five fictional characters known throughout the world; the others are Robin Hood, Tarzan, Mickey Mouse, and Superman (National Public Radio, "Weekend Edition," 28 Feb. 1988, Harlan Ellison.).

27. Most of these tales were told at the Pithotomy Club, a medical student eating club that was founded at Osler's home in 1897 and continues to the present day. The stories were usually easier to swallow than the food.

28. A Garrod. The lessons of rare maladies. *Lancet*. 1928;**I**:1055-60. This is the text of an address that was given before the Medical Society of London. Garrod was Osler's successor as Regius professor at Oxford and coined the phrase "inborn errors of metabolism."

29. WB Bean. *Rare Diseases and Lesions: Their Contributions to Clinical Medicine*. Springfield, Illinois: Thomas; 1967. Foreword by VA McKusick.

30. GM Gould, WL Pyle. *Anomalies and Curiosities of Medicine*. London: Rebman; 1898. Reprinted 1956 by the Julian Press, New York.

31. NS Stern. *Rare Diseases in Internal Medicine.* Springfield, Illinois: Thomas; 1966.

32. FP Weber. *Rare Diseases and Some Debatable Subjects.* Second edition, revised. London: Staples Press; 1947. This book and its successor are astonishing. They clearly reflect the incredible detail with which Weber must have examined his patients. He was prolific as well, publishing roughly 1200 times during his lifetime (and up until a few weeks before his death at age 99). Equally amazing is the number of syndromes that bear his name: Klippel-Trenauny-Weber, Sturge-Weber, Weber-Christian, Osler-Weber-Rendu, Weber-Cockayne (familial recurrent bullous eruption of the hands and feet), and Vaquez-Osler-Weber (polycythemia vera with splenomegaly). (*JAMA*. 1963;**183**:45-9.)

33. FP Weber. *Further Rare Diseases and Debatable Subjects.* London: Staples Press; 1949.

34. J Antionades. *Uncommon Malignant Tumors.* New York: Mason; 1982.

35. JC Birnholz, PE Michelson. *Clinical Diagnostic Pearls.* Flushing, New York: Medical Examination; 1971.

36. A Clain, ed. *Hamilton Bailey's Demonstrations of Physical Signs in Clinical Surgery.* 17th ed. Bristol, UK: Wright; 1986. Though somewhat of a dinosaur in style and content, this is a fascinating book to *read.* It reminds us that physicians once had to made hard decisions without benefit of such conveniences as CT scanning. Bailey shows us how this was done and how the history and physical had to be relied upon.

37. RL DeGowin. *DeGowin & DeGowin's Bedside Diagnostic Examination.* 5th ed. New York: Macmillan; 1987. Another good read.

38. VA McKusick. *Mendelian Inheritance in Man.* 7th ed. Baltimore: Johns Hopkins; 1986. The eighth edition (1988) appeared just as *Zebra Cards* went to press.

39. For example, see: (i) IH Scheinberg. Investigating diseases no one's got. *N Engl J Med.* 1983;**309**:918-9, where the example of Wilson disease is cited; and (ii) WB Shelley, ED Shelley. The orphan patient. *N Engl J Med.* 1988;**318**:646.

40. EA Murphy. *Skepsis, Dogma and Belief.* Baltimore: Johns Hopkins; 1981:68, 157-8.

41. S Dell. Why are classic cases rare? [Letter]. *N Engl J Med.* 1980;**303**:-228.

42. Page 8 of*Further Rare Diseases and Debatable Subjects* (reference 33).

43. A medical Zeno's paradox, in a sense. Of course, more than a few arbitrary decisions about what exactly constitutes "rare" and "disease" would have to be made. As a guideline, however, genetic diseases in aggregate are estimated to affect 1% of all persons (*J Med Genet.* 1977;**14**:316-20) and to account for 5% of pediatric hospital admissions (H Galjaard. *Genetic Metabolic Diseases: Early Diagnosis and Prenatal Analysis.* Amsterdam: Elsevier/North-Holland; 1980:5-38; as cited by: *Mayo Clin Proc.* 1987;**62**:387-404).

44. FH Garrison. *An Introduction to the History of Medicine.* 4th ed. Philadelphia: WB Saunders; 1929:5.

45. However, having just compiled the index and inspected the length of the "sign" entry, the author is forced to admit his considerable chagrin. The many foibles of eponyms are humorously described in: *Perspect Biol Med.* 1979;**22**:170-84.

46. This is discussed in the introduction of *Mendelian Inheritance in Man* (reference 38 above) and in *Ann Intern Med.* 1988;**108**:630-1. I have, alas, bowed to current stylistic dogma and made all syndromic eponyms nonpossessive – but can you really say "Bell palsy" or "Crohn disease" comfortably?

47. S Shem. *The House of God.* New York: Dell; 1978:39.

48. Page 5 of *An Introduction to the History of Medicine* (reference 44).

49. Unfortunately, even an infinite lifespan may be inadequate. Facts are now being generated by biomedical scientists faster than a person can assimilate them: roughly 5500 articles are added to the literature per day (*Ann Intern Med.* 1986;**105**:149-53). The situation is, therefore, similar to the "marching Chinese" scenario popularized early in this century (R Ripley. *Believe It or Not!* New York: Simon and Schuster; 1929:46-7).

50. H Melville. *Moby-Dick.* New York: Norton; 1967:127-8. This is the conclusion of chapter 32, "Cetology."

51. W Osler. The importance of post-graduate study. *Lancet.* 1900;**II**:73-5. The quote also appears in: CNB Camac, ed. *Counsels and Ideals from the Writings of William Osler.* Birmingham, Alabama: Classics of Medicine Library; 1985:70.

52. Most of *Zebra Cards* were written while the author was at Johns Hopkins. Osler, of course, wrote his famous textbook of medicine while at Hopkins, only to have it falter after the 16th edition in 1947 until it was revived by the Hopkins Department of Medicine in 1972. It is not widely known, however, that Osler's successor as physician-in-chief at Hopkins, Llewelys F. Barker, also wrote a textbook. Called *The Clinical Diagnosis of Internal Diseases* (New York: Appleton; 1916),

this three-volume work addressed the use of the history, physical, and laboratory in medical diagnosis. Although the current author has no illusions about his own work, it has appealed to his sense of symmetry to consider *Zebra Cards* as a revival in spirit, if nothing else, of the Barker textbook.

53. G Majno. *The Healing Hand: Man and Wound in the Ancient World.* Cambridge, Massachusetts: Harvard; 1975:1. This fascinating work, written by a pathologist, was a Book-of-the-Month Club selection. (A description of its writing is in *JAMA*. 1982;**247**:2882-4. There is supposedly a second volume on the way.) The quotation appears in the opening paragraph, and suggests how intimately life and healing are linked. Although the literature of medicine spans roughly 4000 years, attempts at healing (in the form of trephination) may have started as early as 10,000 BC.

54. Page 29 of *Bailey* (reference 36). DeGowin and DeGowin report that the term used in Germany is *Augenblick* diagnosis, literally meaning "the blink of an eye" (page 38 of reference 37).

55. FA Willus, TE Keys. *Classics of Cardiology*. Volume 2. New York: Dover; 1961:831-3. This Holmes, a physician, was the father of Supreme Court Justice Holmes.

56. John M. Leonard, MD. National Institutes of Health. 13 April 1981. Leonard, of course, is no longer involved in clinical medicine.

57. As quoted by *DeGowin and DeGowin* (reference 37).

58. F Smithline. Up the Bronchial Tree. *Perspect Biol Med*. 1982;**25**:-436-43. [Copyright ©1982 by the University of Chicago. All rights reserved. Used with permission.]

59. RG Petersdorf. Academic medicine: no longer threadbare or genteel. *N Engl J Med*. 1981;**304**:841-3.

60. Page 24 of *Mnemonics, Rhetorics and Poetics for Medics* (reference 61).

61. RL Bloomfield, ET Chandler. *Mnemonics, Rhetorics and Poetics for Medics*. Winston-Salem, North Carolina; Harbinger Press: 1982:59-60.

62. "The Origin of Sherlock Holmes" is a chapter in: TH Hall. *Sherlock Holmes and his Creator*. New York: St. Martin's Press; 1977:70-90. [Copyright ©1977 by Trevor H. Hall. Used with permission.] This scholarly, well-referenced work is skeptical of recent arguments that Bell was not the primary model for Holmes. These and other Bell stories are (reportedly) in:

    - V Starrett. *The Private Life of Sherlock Holmes*. London; 1934:4-6.

- R Crockett, ed. *Leaves from the Life of a Country Doctor (Clement Bryce Gunn, MD, JP)*. Edinburgh; 1935:35-6. Gunn was a medical student with Doyle.
- WS Baring-Gould. *The Annotated Sherlock Holmes.* New York: Clarkson N. Potter; 1967.
- JME Saxby. *Joseph Bell. MD, FRCS, JP, DL etc. An Appreciation by an Old Friend.* Edinburgh: Oliphant, Anderson and Ferrier; 1913. This rare book has the full story of the deserter.
- AC Doyle. *Memories and Adventures.* London: Hodder and Stoughton; 1924. This is Doyle's autobiography.
- Harold Emery Jones, MD. The Original of Sherlock Holmes. *Colliers Magazine*. 9 January 1904.

63. CBS-TV about 5:30 pm EST on 30 March 1981.

64. Stephen P. Spielberg, MD. Johns Hopkins Hospital. 9 March 1981. This statement represents pediatric dogma.

65. W Osler. Ephemerides. *Montreal Med J.* 1895-1896;**24**:518-9.

66. *Ibid.* Even Flint's voluminous records are exceeded by those of British neurologist Samuel Gowers (1845-1915). His notes on 20,000 personally observed patients fill "hundreds of volumes" despite being written in shorthand! (*Am J Cardiol.* 1989;**63**:241-4).

67. P Beighton, G Beighton. *The Man Behind the Syndrome.* Berlin: Springer-Verlag; 1986:191. This is a collection of biographical sketches of people who have genetic disorders named after them. (It also includes a few women, for example, Gertrud Hurler.) The authors, alas, appear to have somewhat stretched the Weber story as it appeared in his obituary (*Lancet.* 1962;**I**:1308-9). See also *JAMA.* 1963;**183**:45-9.

68. From "A Wish." In: M Arnold. *New Poems.* London: Macmillan; 1867:150-3.

69. Page 15 of *An Introduction to the History of Medicine* (reference 44).

70. *Encyclopædia Britannica.* Volume 16. Chicago: Encyclopædia Britannica, Inc.; 1973:858. This principle, popularly known as "Ockham's razor," may be translated as: "Multiplicity ought not be posited without necessity."

71. Quoted on page 15 of *An Introduction to the History of Medicine* (reference 44). La Rouchefoucald (1613-1680) was a French classical author who treated the *maxime* as a literary form.

72. Page 7 of *An Introduction to the History of Medicine* (reference 44).

73. AM Harvey, J Boardley. *Differential Diagnosis.* 2nd ed. Philadelphia: WB Saunders; 1970:787. Dr. Harvey was not in the habit of making incorrect diagnoses, and did not do so in this case.

74. F Adams (transl). *The Genuine Works of Hippocrates.* Huntington, New York: Robert E. Krieger; 1972:17-8. This is paragraph 23 of the book *On Ancient Medicine.*

75. AM Harvey, et al. *Differential Diagnosis.* 3rd ed. Philadelphia: WB Saunders; 1979:15.

76. Such unusual statements appear to this day in the medical literature, for example, "routine indications [for a pacemaker] may be the rule, but exceptional cases are not rare" (*N Engl J Med.* 1988;**318**:182-3). The way medical professionals evaluate qualitative expressions of probability is discussed in: *N Engl J Med.* 1986;**315**:740-4.

77. As quoted by Garrod (reference 28).

78. RB Bean, WB Bean. *Sir William Osler: Aphorisms from his Bedside Teachings and Writings.* New York: Henry Schuman; 1950:128. Out of print, unfortunately.

79. Page 4 of *The Effective Clinician* (reference 82). You can also try *N Engl J Med.* 1970;**283**:20-4, which is the first chapter of the book.

80. *Omni Magazine.* March 1981:126.

81. Page 93 of *Aphorisms* (reference 78).

82. PA Tumulty. *The Effective Clinician.* Philadelphia: WB Saunders; 1973:3. The first half of this book is an education that can now be obtained nowhere else: Tumulty's pearls about how to interact with patients and their families. This book cannot be recommended too highly. Sadly, it is out of print, but most medical libraries should have it. (A derivative of the title lives on, however, in Harrell & Firestein's popular book for medical students, *The Effective Scutboy* (reference 13). They were both pupils of "The Tums" at Johns Hopkins.)

83. H Zinsser. *Rats, Lice and History.* Boston: Little, Brown; 1934:167. A delightful "biography" of typhus. As for Beyle, he is not listed in my edition of *Encyclopædia Britannica.*

84. DE Knuth. *Sorting and Searching.* (Volume 3 of *The Art of Computer Programming.*) Reading, Massachusetts: Addison-Wesley; 1973:723. The quotation is particularly apropos to this index; astute readers will notice some small peculiarities of alphabetization.

The Protein Tree of the Genus <u>Equus</u>

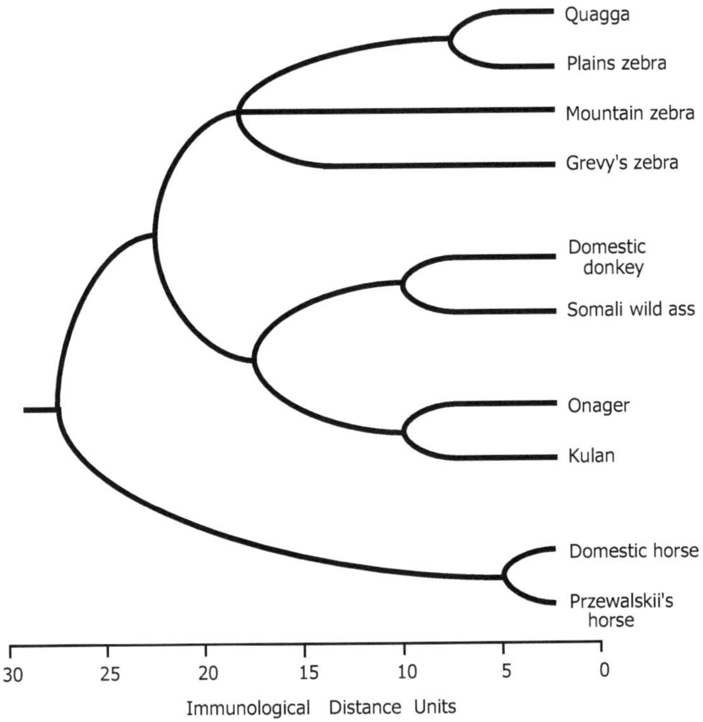

(Adapted with permission from *Experientia.* 1985;**41**:1192-3.)

Harvey's Precepts

Transcribed (more or less accurately) from a March 1983 lecture

1. Never miss an opportunity to examine a patient. – W. S. Thayer
   - The more you see, the better.
   - Enables you to develop a standardized approach.

2. Develop your techniques of gaining rapport with the patient.
   - Present to the patient his or her image of what a physician should be, not *your* image.
   - That is, look and act like a doctor.

3. Collection and analysis of information proceed in parallel.
   - For example, the questions you ask when taking a history depend on the answers to previous questions.

4. Only through practice can you separate normal from abnormal, relevant from irrelevant.

5. The most common errors of interpretation are those of overinterpretation.
   - New information should generate new hypotheses, not be assigned to old hypotheses.

6. Always remember you are usually functioning in an atmosphere of calculated uncertainty.
   - You must therefore make decisions before all the evidence is in.
   - Don't procrastinate in these situations.

7. Mistakes should be aired so they can help prevent future errors.
   - Common situations where mistakes occur:
     - When you do not have all the evidence. Avoid this by being thorough.
     - Falling in love with your initial hypothesis.
     - Failure to recognize that illnesses are not static, that they progress. Write a progress note when you re-evaluate your thinking in a complex illness; that way the information is in front of you, so you can sit back and take stock of it.

→ Harvey is Dr. A. McGhee Harvey.

8. Keep your medical knowledge current.
   - Every new patient should teach you something.
   - Read the literature; go to conferences.

9. Like what you're doing.
   - Medicine is interesting, competent people of integrity in an atmosphere that is less confrontational than other fields.

10. Know your limitations.
    - Carry a problem to the point where you need consultation.
    - Do not confuse pride with self-respect.

McKusick's Commandments

I Thou shalt avoid becoming a technocrat for whom patients are merely dehumanized objects for application of thy powerful new diagnostic and therapeutic tools.

II Thou shalt honor the memory of thy professional forebears, especially the one for whom thy firm is named.

III Thou shalt attend Medical Grand Rounds regularly.

IV Thou shalt not use eponyms in vain (that is, without knowing the origins thereof).

V Thou shalt wear thy Osler tie/scarf each Friday (but only on Friday), and shalt practice its motto AEQUANIMITAS seven days a week.

VI Thou shalt deliver (not read) thy oral case presentations, prepared in a logical, precise, and concise format.

VII Thou shalt approach the problems of each of thy patients in a scholarly manner in order that thou may do best by thy patient and most for the advancement of medicine.

VIII Thou shalt not covet thy neighbor's split-level house, thou shalt not covet thy neighbor's swimming pool, nor thy neighbor's Mercedes, nor thy neighbor's Acapulco vacation, lest thou yield to the temptation to moonlight.

IX Thou shalt laugh WITH thy patient and thy fellow health professionals, and, whenever appropriate, AT thyself, and shall maintain a smile even under the most difficult circumstances.

X Thou shalt honor thy ACS [Assistant Chief of Service] and tell everyone of his or her great sagacity, humanity, and clinical acumen.

→ McKusick is Dr. Victor McKusick.

The Principles and Practices of Internship

Composed 1985 by (slightly paranoid) former interns

1. Talk to your patients.
2. Your first job is to get them better.
3. Look at your scut sheet.
   - You do not go home until *everything* is crossed off.
   - Never go home without signing out pending laboratory results.
4. Write it down unless you *want* to forget it.
   - If you've been told twice, you've erred.
5. You are not supervised as closely as you think.
   - You can only get in trouble for *not* asking.
6. Excuses don't help patients.
7. Never trust emergency room diagnoses.
   - Completely re-assess the patient yourself.
8. If you want it done right, do it yourself.
9. Would you trust Escort with *your* CSF?
   - Hand deliver all body fluids.
10. Never refuse a hit.
    - Let your resident try to do it.
11. Smile in the Acc.
    - Never show your face in the Accident room unless you are there to get a patient.
12. Don't let a patient crash on you alone.
    - Call your resident or call a consultant.
13. Trust no one.

In Summary:

- Keep them alive until morning.
- Order the studies, chart the results, let others worry about fancy interpretations.
- Cover your ass.

Listing of Cards

Abdomen

AB-001	umbilical position
AB-002	blue umbilicus
AB-003	splenomegaly and dialysis
AB-004	periumbilical macules
AB-005	vein from groin to axilla
AB-006	flank discolorations
AB-007	umbilical nodule
AB-008	radiopaque medications

Blood

BL-001	bleeding after transfusion
BL-002	acquired sickle-cell trait
BL-003	spirochetes on smear
BL-004	clotted purple-top tube
BL-005	bright red venous blood
BL-006	thrombocytopenia?

Diet

DI-001	pain after drinking alcohol
DI-002	weakness after spaghetti
DI-003	immobility after protein
DI-004	pellagra
DI-005	protein-induced headaches
DI-006	paper pica
DI-007	red urine after eating beets
DI-008	return of pregnancy's cravings

Ear

EA-001 ear lobe creases
EA-002 vertigo and tragus pressing
EA-003 referred ear pain
EA-004 buzzing above the head
EA-005 bullous myringitis
EA-006 calcified pinnae
EA-007 ear inflammation sparing the lobe
EA-008 exostoses of external auditory canal
EA-009 hypesthesia of the external auditory canal
EA-010 ear lobe spots

Endocrine

EN-001 normoglycemic hypoglycemia

Extremities

EX-001 hot weather limb pains
EX-002 hot weather limb pains, sort of

Hands and Feet

EX-201 high arches
EX-202 wide toe spacing
EX-203 toe autoamputation
EX-204 toe bullae
EX-205 skin nonwrinkling in water

Lower

EX-401 venous stasis in men
EX-402 anterior bowing of tibias
EX-403 sneezing and leg pain
EX-404 orthostatic leg itching
EX-405 can run but not walk
EX-406 adolescent knee effusions
EX-407 thigh/buttock ringed rash

Upper

EX-601 hairy elbows

Eye

EY-001 poor vision in a hot shower
EY-002 pulsatile unilateral exophthalmos

Appendages

EY-201 periorbital purpura

External
- EY-401 pigmented corneal rings
- EY-402 unilateral arcus senilis
- EY-403 brown plaques by the limbus
- EY-404 unilateral scleral icterus

Motor
- EY-601 eyelid twitch
- EY-602 infrequent blinking
- EY-603 persistent nystagmus
- EY-604 eye movements and light flashes

Ophthalmoscopic
- EY-801 pigmented vessel-like streaks

Family History
- FA-001 congenital heart block
- FA-002 adenopathy in families
- FA-003 family history of drowning
- FA-004 everyone at home has the flu

General
- GE-000 great imitators
- GE-001 general classification of disorders
- GE-002 medicine and metal detectors
- GE-003 nonaneurysmal pulsations
- GE-004 micrographia
- GE-005 situs inversus
- GE-006 fishy body odor
- GE-007 both hands on the steering wheel
- GE-008 heroin that burns when injected

GI
- GI-001 silver stools
- GI-002 vomitus categories
- GI-003 pruritus ani
- GI-004 melodic flatulence
- GI-005 seagulls in stool
- GI-006 stool flushing difficulties
- GI-007 vomitus that etches glass
- GI-008 childhood car-sickness

GU
- GU-001 synpharyngitic macroscopic hematuria
- GU-002 pulsatile cervix
- GU-003 left testicular and scrotal swelling

GU-004	post-coital collapse
GU-005	sudden collapse during pregnancy
GU-006	male endometrial carcinoma
GU-007	eosinophiluria
GU-008	penile pain and altered mental status
GU-009	penile horn
GU-010	urine stain darkened by washing
GU-011	micturition headache

Head

HD-001	head clicking
HD-002	rhythmic head nodding
HD-003	adult fontanelle

Face

HD-301	non-wrinkling forehead
HD-302	discharging chin sinus
HD-303	infant's mother's cheek
HD-304	looking younger in Mexico
HD-305	aerophobia
HD-306	hyperpigmented forehead nodules
HD-307	numb chin

Heart

HE-001	weak beat after a premature ventricular contraction
HE-002	pacemaker failure during surgery
HE-003	tumors and congenital cyanosis
HE-004	post-palpitation polyuria
HE-005	sweating in pulmonary edema
HE-006	RV dilatation
HE-007	mental status in the coronary care unit
HE-008	occlusion of large arteries in endocarditis
HE-009	tricky drug levels after myocardial infarction
HE-010	murmur and defenestration
HE-011	severe chest pain

Auscultation

HE-301	loud cardiac sounds
HE-302	dove-coo murmur
HE-303	right parasternal diastolic murmur

EKG

HE-601	flat-line EKG
HE-602	orthostatic normalization of ischemic EKG
HE-603	switching limb leads normalizes EKG
HE-604	progressive PR shortening

Immunology and Infection

IM-001 rubor et tumor cum calore et dolore
IM-002 flu in a welder
IM-003 contact anaphylaxis
IM-004 S. bovis bacteremia
IM-005 two disseminated neisserial infections

Lung

LU-001 pseudohemoptysis
LU-002 sinopulmonary infections and infertility
LU-003 extended breath-holding
LU-004 Pseudomonas bronchitis
LU-005 eosinophilic pleural effusions
LU-006 tri-layered sputum
LU-007 orthostatic dyspnea

Mouth

MO-001 orange tonsils
MO-002 jaw claudication
MO-003 grooves radiating from mouth corners
MO-004 black lip spots

Teeth and Gums

MO-701 notched incisors
MO-702 lipstick on teeth
MO-703 prominent fillings
MO-704 blue gum line

Tongue

MO-801 touching tongue to nose

Musculoskeleton

MU-001 stooped posture
MU-002 bone metastases
MU-003 rapid onset of exertional myalgia
MU-004 arthralgias and breast scars

Neck

NC-001 reduplicated right carotid pulse
NC-002 beauty and the thyroid
NC-003 bounding carotid pulse
NC-004 dipping trachea
NC-005 midline mass that moves with tongue
NC-006 small 7th cervical lymph node

Neuro

NE-001	black cerebrospinal fluid
NE-002	delayed reflex relaxation
NE-003	cerebrospinal fluid that clots
NE-004	anisocoria and coma
NE-005	eyelid tone in coma
NE-006	Babinski caveat
NE-007	CNS symptoms during exercise

Mental status

NE-501	The Tell-Tale Heart
NE-502	post-partum mentality

Nose

NO-001	bifid nasal tip
NO-002	sexual sneezing
NO-003	pruritic nostrils

Skin

SK-001	localized hirsutism
SK-002	sudden appearance of seborrheic keratoses
SK-003	postexertional skin thickening
SK-004	expanding annular lesion
SK-005	pigmentation over blood vessels
SK-006	giant reactions to insect bites
SK-007	warfarin skin necrosis
SK-008	immunity from bedsores
SK-009	skin pustule after sterile pinprick
SK-010	white halo around a mole

Hair

SK-301	frequent beauty parlor visits
SK-302	full head of hair in a man
SK-303	woman lacking axillary and pubic hair

Nails

SK-601	yellow nails and leg edema
SK-602	peri-ungual pigmentation

Thorax

TH-001	butterfly shaped hypopigmentation on the back
TH-002	collar burn rosette
TH-003	suprasternal fat
TH-004	interscapular bruit
TH-005	unilateral clavicular thickening

TH-006 axillary tattoo
TH-007 shoulder pain in the Trendelenburg position
TH-008 paraspinal mass in anemia
TH-009 pulsatile sternoclavicular joint
TH-010 menses and chest pain
TH-011 axillary freckling

Breast

TH-201 areolar papules
TH-202 unilateral gynecomastia

Vital Signs

VI-001 high fever and slow pulse
VI-002 shock and bullae

Temperature

VI-701 fever, headache, and myalgia
VI-702 episodic hypothermia
VI-703 picking at the covers when febrile
VI-704 fever near an airport

Wish List

WI-001 wish list

Index

All books cited in the cards are indexed by title name. Most eponyms are indexed under the "sign" entry; eponymous entities that are not signs are indexed under the individual's last name. Only the cards are indexed.

B

C

F

I

M

N

O

P

S

U

V

W

X

Y

Z

Zebra Cards

Zebra Cards ™

John G. Sotos, M.D.

Formerly of:

Department of Medicine
Johns Hopkins University School of Medicine
Baltimore, Maryland

Abdomen AB-001

Downward displacement of the umbilicus

Abdomen AB-002

Bluish tinge to peri-umbilical skin

The equation

$$a^n + b^n = c^n$$

has solutions in positive integers a, b, c, and n only when $n = 2$ (and there are infinitely many triplets a, b, c which satisfy the equation); but there are no solutions for $n > 2$. I have discovered a truly marvelous proof of this statement, which, unfortunately, this margin is too small to contain.

Pierre de Fermat
(1601[?] – 1665)

(Tanyol sign[1])

* *ascites*

In infants, the distance between the navel and pubis is small relative to body height. During growth the navel migrates superiorly, advancing the furthest in whites, intermediate in Asians, and "not very far at all" in blacks. (Amazingly, this fact was used *circa* 1860 to "document" alleged white superiority and black inferiority.)[2]

Perhaps not bearing that caveat in mind, Bailey states that the normal umbilicus is almost equidistant between the xiphoid and symphysis pubis. It is displaced upwards by swelling arising from the pelvis (for example, pregnancy, ovarian cysts) and downwards by ascites.[1,3] He also notes: "Every time an abdomen is examined the eyes of the clinician, almost instinctively, rest momentarily on the umbilicus. How innumerable are the variations of this structure!"[1]

(1) Hamilton Bailey's Demonstrations of Physical Signs in Clinical Surgery. 17th ed. A Clain (ed). Bristol, UK: Wright (1986). pp 251-252.
(2) The Mismeasure of Man. SJ Gould. New York: Norton (1981). p 40.
(3) It seems reasonable to assume that the Tanyol sign appears only with large amounts of ascites.

(Cullen sign[1,2])
(umbilical black eye[3])

* *ruptured ectopic pregnancy*
* *hemorrhagic pancreatitis*
* *ruptured aortic aneurysm*

When this sign occurs, it is a reliable indication that free blood is present in the retroperitoneum (also see cards AB-006 and TH-007).

Cullen, who was neither the first to observe nor report this sign,[4] had correctly interpreted it before he operated on his index patient. He remembered that a Dr. Joseph Ransohoff of Cincinnati had had a patient with umbilical jaundice who, at surgery, had a large amount of free bile in the abdomen secondary to rupture of the common bile duct.[2] (A yellow peri-umbilical tinge has also been seen in acute pancreatitis.[3])

An abdominal discoloration resembling livedo reticularis has also been observed in acute pancreatitis (Walzel sign),[4] as has staining below the inguinal ligament (Fox sign).[5]

Ecchymoses from a leaking aorta may appear at just about any site; *viz*, a ruptured abdominal aortic aneurysm can stain the skin anywhere from the umbilicus to the knee.[6]

(1) Am J Obstet. **78**: 457 only (1918). Cullen's description.
(2) Johns Hopkins Med J. **137**: 224-234 (1975). Historical aspects of the discovery.
(3) Hamilton Bailey's Demonstrations of Physical Signs in Clinical Surgery. 17th ed. A Clain (ed). Bristol, UK: Wright (1986). p 256. Illustration.
(4) New Engl J Med. **251**: 851-853 (1954). Cutaneous signs of acute pancreatitis.
(5) Surgical Diagnosis. G Quist. London: HK Lewis (1977). p 283. Cited by reference 4.
(6) J Emerg Med. **5**: 323-329 (1987). Nice discussion of ruptured abdominal aortic aneurysms.

Abdomen AB-003

Splenomegaly in a hemodialysis patient

Abdomen AB-004

Punctate dark blue macules
around the umbilicus

Abdomen AB-005

Visible vein,
extending from inguinal region to axilla

* *silicone accumulation in spleen*[1,2]

The silicone was torn off the dialysis tubing by the action of the roller pumps. Pancytopenia, also present in the index patient, responded to splenectomy.[1]

Although silicone is chemically stable and rarely excites an immunologic reaction from the body, several hazards associated with its use have been reported recently:

- acute pneumonitis – after subcutaneous injection in three transsexual men;[3]
- granulomatous hepatitis – has occurred after both breast augmentation and after damage to the silicone ball of a Starr-Edwards prosthetic heart valve;[3]
- hypercalcemia – silicone-induced granulomas may secrete calcitriol, much like sarcoid granulomas do;[4]
- syncope – a woman's pacemaker migrated into her augmentation mammoplasty prosthesis and stopped working;[5]
- further hazards as noted on card MU-004.

(1) New Engl J Med. **305**: 1077-1079 (1981). Case report.
(2) New Engl J Med. **306**: 135-140; **307**: 319-320 (1982). Accumulation in liver, spleen, and other organs. Of course, there are many other causes of organomegaly in dialysis patients.
(3) Lancet. **II**: 833 only (1983). Editorial on the hazards of silicone.
(4) New Engl J Med. **311**: 1103-1105 (1984). Editorial: calcium, calcitriol, & granulomatous disease.
(5) New Engl J Med. **303**: 817 only (1980). Letter. "Silicone syncope."

---

* *Fabry Disease*[1] *(alpha-galactosidase A deficiency)*

These lesions begin as punctate dark-blue, red, or black nonblanching macules. Often diagnosed as petechiae, they are angiokeratomas.[2] Most frequently they lie in a "bathing suit" distribution and tend to cluster around the umbilicus, on the scrotum, and over pressure points. Often difficult to spot in childhood, there is a progressive increase in the size and number of lesions with age. As individual lesions enlarge to 1 to 2 mm, they may blanch or be slightly raised.[1]

Fabry disease is an X-linked disorder of glycosphingolipid metabolism affecting virtually every organ in the body (McKusick 30150). Common presentations in young men include acroparesthesias (card EX-001), "petechiae," heat intolerance, unexplained hyperpyrexia, or proteinuria. Heterozygous females are affected with varying degrees of severity. Slit lamp examination may show the typical "propeller" shaped opacities in the lenses. Biochemical diagnosis rests on demonstrating decreased alpha galactosidase activity in plasma, leukocytes, or tissue.[1]

Angiokeratomas are seen in other lysosomal storage disorders, including fucosidosis and a form of sialidase deficiency. Fordyce lesions (benign scrotal angiokeratomas in older men) and angiokeratoma circumscripta must also be excluded.[1]

(1) The Metabolic Basis of Inherited Disease. 5th ed. JB Stanbury et al (eds). New York: McGraw-Hill (1983). pp 906-944. Exhaustive treatment; is updated and condensed in: TB Fitzpatrick et al. Dermatology in General Medicine. 3rd ed. New York: McGraw-Hill (1987). pp 1739-1760.
(2) That is, angiectases with thin vascular walls and minimal hyperkeratosis of the overlying skin.

---

* *obstruction of the inferior vena cava (IVC)*

Inguino-axillary veins must be present bilaterally to diagnose IVC obstruction; unilateral presence of such a vein suggests blockage of the ipsilateral common- or external-iliac vein.[1a]

IVC obstruction can also lead to collateral flow through dilated superficial abdominal vessels. These may be seen within a week of complete obstruction; using red goggles facilitates their visualization. DeGowin & DeGowin discuss how the visible pattern of collateralization helps localize the anatomic site of the obstruction.[2]

Portal hypertension and/or portal obstruction are other causes of dilated superficial abdominal veins (the famous "caput medusa"). To distinguish a caput from the dilated superficial veins of IVC obstruction, examine the direction of flow in the veins inferior to the umbilicus. Normally the veins inferior to the umbilicus flow inferiorly, and those superior to it, superiorly. Portal hypertension has no effect on this. However, with IVC obstruction, flow in the veins inferior to the umbilicus will be reversed, as blood is shunted through superficial veins to the superior vena cava.[1b,3]

(1) Hamilton Bailey's Demonstrations of Physical Signs in Clinical Surgery. 17th ed. A Clain (ed). Bristol, UK: Wright (1986). [a] pp 18-19; illustrated. [b] pp 249-250; illustrated.
(2) DeGowin & DeGowin's Bedside Diagnostic Examination. 5th ed. RL DeGowin. New York: Macmillan (1987). pp 452-453.
(3) Bean warns that since there are no venous valves in newly developed collaterals, determining the direction of blood flow can be difficult. [Rare Diseases and Lesions. WB Bean. Springfield, IL: Thomas (1967). pp 161-163.]

Abdomen AB-006

Bilateral loin or flank discolorations
of a dirty greenish color

Abdomen AB-007

Firm, indurated plaque or nodule
at the umbilicus

Abdomen AB-008

Abdominal x-ray showing radiopaque material
in the stomach or bowel

(Grey Turner sign[1,2])

* *hemorrhagic pancreatitis*
* *ruptured aortic aneurysm*
* *ruptured ectopic pregnancy*

Both the Grey Turner sign and the Cullen sign (card AB-002) are thought to result from the tracking of blood-stained retroperitoneal fluid through the tissues of the abdominal wall or along the falciform ligament to the umbilical area. We will refer to them collectively as body wall ecchymoses (BWE).

In a series of 23 patients with BWE (representing 3% of 770 consecutive patients hospitalized for pancreatitis), the mean age was 56 (range, 20 to 83); 75% were women, and all major causes of pancreatitis were represented. BWE appeared most commonly on the fourth hospital day (range, 2 to 6); 40% had the Cullen sign, 40% the Grey Turner, and 20% had both.[3]

By objective criteria, 87% of those with BWE had "severe" pancreatitis, and 96% suffered "serious" complications; 37% died, but the presence of BWE was not an independent risk factor for death. Age, however, was important: Those with BWE who were under age 54 all survived, while those over 70 all died soon after the sign appeared. Of those surviving longer than 5 days, 37% developed pseudocysts.[3]

(1) Br J Surg. **7**: 394-395 (1919). Turner's original description. (Grey was his middle name.)
(2) JAMA. **247**: 2754 only (1982). Large color photo.
(3) Surg Gynecol Obstet. **159**: 343-347 (1984). Study from Scotland.
Also see card TH-007.

(Sister Mary Joseph nodule[1,2])

* *cancer, metastatic to the umbilicus*

Sister Mary Joseph, onetime first surgical assistant to W. J. Mayo, is generally credited as the first to appreciate the ominous prognostic significance of metastases to the umbilicus: Most patients die within 10 months after the nodule appears.[2] A recent study from her institution (the Mayo clinic) reported 85 cases occurring over 32 years: 45 in women and 40 in men. Ages ranged from 32 to 91 and averaged 61. In 45 of the 85 the umbilical lesion developed within 12 months of the diagnosis of the internal malignancy; in 12 it was the initial presentation. Clinically, the nodule is seen as a firm, indurated plaque or nodule, usually with a vascular appearance.[2]

In 50% of the cases a primary gastrointestinal cancer was found (stomach 20%, colon 14%, pancreas 11%, small bowel 5%, gallbladder <1%). Female reproductive cancers accounted for 27% of *all* primaries (ovary 14%, endometrium 5%, breast 5%, cervix <1%). Prostate and lung primaries occurred once, and 20% of primaries were unknown.[2]

Metastases can reach the umbilicus by contiguous extension from the peritoneal surface, by hematogenous spread as with any cutaneous metastasis, or by spread along various anatomic structures near the umbilicus. Beware, however: A concretion, pilonidal cyst, hypertrophic scar/keloid, hernia, benign tumor, focus of endometriosis, or other lesion may present as an umbilical nodule.[2]

(1) New Engl J Med. **316**: 1348-1349; **317**: 902 only (1987). Was Sister Joseph's first name Mary?
(2) J Am Acad Dermatol. **10**: 610-615 (1984). Clinical and histologic study. Says it was Mary.

---

* *phenothiazines, tricyclic antidepressants*
* *metals (arsenic, lead, iron)*
* *enteric coated medications (salicylates, potassium chloride)*
* *iodides, chlorides (carbon tetrachloride, chloroform, chloral hydrate)*

In a study of 211 solid medications,[1] 15% were moderately radiopaque, 4% were markedly so, and 1% to 2% were densely radiopaque. Of the medications at least moderately radiopaque, 20% disintegrated in gastric juice in less than 20 minutes, 40% between 20 and 120 minutes, and 40% remained intact for 2 hours.

Radiopacity can be related to the medication itself; to its vehicle, binder, or formulation technique; or to any combination of these factors. Enteric-coated medications tend to be radiopaque, as do medications containing atoms of high atomic weight (for example, heavy metals and iodides). Of the major drugs with abuse potential, only the phenothiazines and tricyclic antidepressants possess moderate radiopacity.[2]

(1) Clin Radiol. **98**: 525-533 (1971). Study of 211 medications.
(2) Goldfrank's Toxicologic Emergencies. 3rd ed. L Goldfrank et al (eds). Norwalk, CT: Appleton-Century-Crofts (1986). pp 53-55, 615-617.
(–) Health-food faddists may have radiopaque bone meal fragments in the abdomen and/or pelvis [AJR: Am J Roentgenol. **130**: 789-790 (1978).].
(–) Zinc and bismuth lend radiopacity to suppositories [Radiology. **121**: 71-73 (1976).].

Blood BL-001

Bleeding one week after a blood transfusion

Blood BL-002

Acquired sickle-cell trait

Blood BL-003

Spirochete seen on the blood smear
of a febrile patient

** post-transfusion purpura due to anti-platelet antibodies*

Red cell products (other than washed or frozen/thawed erythrocytes) also contain platelets or platelet fragments. These can lead to immunization against, then destruction of, the recipient's platelets. Ninety-eight percent of people have platelet antigen PL^{A1}. If $PL^{A1}(+)$ platelets enter a $PL^{A1}(-)$ patient who has been sensitized to PL^{A1} antigen (for example, by previous transfusion or by pregnancy), an antibody against the antigen is raised after about a week, and the transfused platelets are destroyed.

How the recipient's native platelets are destroyed is uncertain. It may be an "innocent bystander" effect, where immune complexes of antibody and $PL^{A1}(+)$ transfused platelets become attached to the native platelets and lead to their destruction. Another theory rests on the fact that platelets are known to acquire antigens on their surface by absorption: If PL^{A1} antigen eluted from the transfused platelets were adsorbed onto the native platelets, it would make them a target for the antibody.

In any case, the thrombocytopenia is profound and persists for several weeks.

(–) Blood. **45**: 529-536 (1975). Report of three cases.
(–) Mayo Clin Proc. **57**: 778-780 (1982). Laboratory considerations.
(–) New Engl J Med. **318**: 500-508 (1988). CPC on post-transfusion purpura, with a nice discussion of pathophysiology.

** blood transfusion*

If a blood donor has sickle trait, then hemoglobin S (HbS) will be passed to the transfusion recipient. This iatrogenic sickle-cell "trait" can be identified by the small percentage of HbS found on hemoglobin electrophoresis (5% in the patient reported in the reference) or by the low proportion of cells that sickle with the metabisulfate test.

New Engl J Med. **306**: 1487 only (1982). Letter.

** relapsing fever*[1]

A variety of *Borrelia* species may cause relapsing fever. However, unlike the other spirochetes that cause human disease (the treponemes and leptospires), they are readily stained by the Giemsa or Wright procedure.[2]

Tick-borne relapsing fever is the only form of the disease in the United States, occurring sporadically during the summer in mountainous Western areas. After a 7-day incubation, illness begins abruptly with high fever, shaking chills, and severe headache, followed by prostration, myalgias, abdominal pain, vomiting, and cough.[2]

High fever (39.4 to 40.6°C) persists for 3 to 6 days, until the characteristic crisis of defervescence occurs (a sudden fall in temperature accompanied by drenching sweats). Spirochetes are rapidly cleared from the blood and the patient remains afebrile until 6 to 10 days later when mutated organisms appear in the blood in what may be the first of several relapses.[2]

Of patients with "Borreliosis," 25% to 50% will have visible spirochetes; a positive finding is highly specific.[3] Repeated examinations may be necessary to demonstrate the organism, which is not seen in the blood during the afebrile intervals.[2]

(1) Infectious Diseases. (Pocket Picture Guides to Clinical Medicine) WE Farrar & HP Lambert. Baltimore: Williams & Wilkins (1984). p 52. Illustrated. The American and African Trypanosomes have a spiral shape and may also appear on smears (p 70).
(2) "Leptospirosis, relapsing fever, rat-bite fever, and Lyme disease." In: Scientific American Medicine. E Rubenstein & DD Federman (eds). New York: Scientific American (2/88). 7:VII:3-5. Illust.
(3) Medical Microbiology and Infectious Diseases. A Braude. Philadelphia: Saunders (1981). pp 490-5.
(–) Laboratory Diagnosis of Infectious Diseases. A Balows et al. New York: Springer (1988). pp 105-110.

Blood BL-004

Inability to draw a blood sample
without having it clot in the tube

Blood BL-005

Bright red venous blood

Blood BL-006

Thrombocytopenia reported from the laboratory,
but
normal number of platelets on smear

* *severe hypercalcemia*

To prevent clotting of the specimen, conventional "purple top" phlebotomy tubes contain EDTA. This chemical chelates calcium, thereby interrupting the clotting cascade before it ever gets started. A patient with a serum calcium level of 20.4 mg/dL (who was, incidentally, asymptomatic) had enough calcium in his blood to both saturate the EDTA and trigger the clotting cascade in the sample tube.[1]

Intrinsic blood disease may cause similar results. In rare cases of paraproteinemia, use of a Butterfly* needle to draw blood may result in clotting while use of a Vacutainer may not.[2]

(1) New Engl J Med. **307**: 684-685 (1982). Letter.
(2) William R. Bell, MD; Johns Hopkins Hospital; November 1983. Possible mechanism(s) could depend on some property of the Butterfly's plastic tubing or on a temperature effect.
(*) Registered trademark.

---

* *carbon monoxide poisoning*
* *hydrogen cyanide poisoning*

When carbon monoxide combines with hemoglobin, carboxyhemoglobin is formed. This stable, cherry-red compound[1] imparts a bright red color to blood, which is an important clue to the presence of carbon monoxide poisoning.[2] Uncommonly, skin, mucous membranes, and finger nails assume a cherry color as well.[2]

Hydrogen cyanide causes histotoxic hypoxia. That is, the cytochrome chain in mitochondria is poisoned, and peripheral tissues become unable to utilize oxygen. Thus, peripheral oxygen tensions rise, removing the concentration gradient that normally powers the dissociation of O_2 from oxyhemoglobin. The result is a high venous concentration of bright red oxyhemoglobin.[2,3,4] Hydrogen sulfide poisoning displays a similar chemistry.[3]

Distinguishing these poisons is crucial because their treatments are different.[2] Bright red blood is frequently absent in both (even in severe poisoning),[2] and standard arterial blood gas measurements of PaO_2 are usually normal, as this technique measures only the O_2 dissolved in plasma.[1]

(1) Medical Physiology. 14th ed. VB Mountcastle (ed). St. Louis: Mosby (1980). pp 1921-1924.
(2) Goldfrank's Toxicologic Emergencies. 3rd ed. L Goldfrank et al (eds). Norwalk, CT: Appleton-Century-Crofts (1986). Carbon monoxide is covered on pp 662-668, cyanide on pp 585-593.
(3) Casarett and Doull's Toxicology. CD Klaassen et al. New York: Macmillan (1986). pp 240-242.
(4) High venous oxygen levels will make arteries and veins appear similar in the ocular fundus.
(–) Shock and/or tissue death reduces peripheral oxygen extraction; arteriovenous fistulae locally brighten venous blood.

(pseudo-thrombocytopenia)

* *spurious laboratory result, due to artifactual clumping of platelets*

Platelet clumps cannot be properly counted by automated blood analyzers: Some clumps will be ignored and others may be counted as leukocytes. This results in pseudo-thrombocytopenia and occasionally pseudo-leukocytosis.[1]

The clumping is apparently due to immunoglobulins, triggered by the anticoagulants found in conventional phlebotomy tubes (and/or by a temperature drop).[1] For example, some patients have anti-platelet antibodies that interact with platelets only in the absence of calcium.[2] Calcium absence does not occur in vivo, but does in a "purple top" phlebotomy tube containing the calcium-chelating anticoagulant EDTA (card BL-004). Heparin and sodium citrate cause platelet clumping less often than EDTA.[1]

Up to 1 in 50 of ill, hospitalized patients have EDTA-induced platelet clumping.[3] Some automated blood analyzers attempt to detect the presence of these clumps, but no one has yet suggested relying solely on this ability.[1,3] Thus, examination of a *finger-stick* blood smear *must* be done before labelling a patient thrombocytopenic.[4] The consequences of an incorrect diagnosis are potentially disastrous.[2,5]

(1) Am J Clin Pathol. **89**: 634-639 (1988). Pseudo-thrombocytopenia with various anticoagulants.
(2) New Engl J Med. **318**: 500-508 (1988). CPC on thrombocytopenia.
(3) Mayo Clin Proc. **59**: 123-125 (1984). Nice review of pseudo-thrombocytopenia.
(4) Or leukopenic or leukocytotic. Also, platelet counts are artifactually lowered in polycythemia (centrifuged red cell ghosts pull platelets down to the tube bottom with them).
(5) Scand J Haematol. **37**: 341-346 (1986). Horror stories.

Diet DI-001

Pain after drinking alcohol

Diet DI-002

Thirty-year-old Asian man
with generalized weakness
after a spaghetti meal
in December

Diet DI-003

Patient eats a high-protein meal,
then cannot move

* *tumor*

* *osteomyelitis, sarcoidosis, pancreatitis, simple fractures, normal subjects*

Pain is but one manifestation of the syndrome of alcohol intolerance that sometimes accompanies the development of neoplasia. Other manifestations of alcohol intolerance are bleeding, vomiting, headache, dyspnea, decreased intoxication threshold, loss of desire for alcohol, and sudden dislike for its taste. Not uncommonly, part of the syndrome will precede all other symptoms of neoplasia.[1,2]

Occasionally generalized, the pain is usually felt at the site of the tumor minutes after a drink. Patients with Hodgkin disease and other lymphomas may have alcohol intolerance in 20% to 40% of cases. Carcinoma of the cervix, bladder, lung, and other tumors cause it less often.[1,2]

One man with recurrent Hodgkin disease had supraclavicular pain after eating spicy foods such as pizza or Mexican-food TV-dinners.[3]

(Because ethanol induces the liver's cytochrome P-450 enzyme system,[4] it may precipitate an acute neurovascular attack in patients with one of the hepatic porphyrias.[5])

(1) AJR: Am J Roentgenol. **64**: 913-918 (1950). Original description.
(2) Br Med J. **2**: 437-441 (1966). Interesting review of this topic; supplies the differential listed.
(3) New Engl J Med. **287**: 203 only (1972). Mexican TV dinner pain.
(4) Ann Intern Med. **104**: 427-429 (1986). Alcohol and cytochrome P-450 (and acetaminophen).
(5) Cecil Textbook of Medicine. 16th ed. JB Wyngaarden & LH Smith Jr (eds). Philadelphia: Saunders (1982). pp 1123-1125.

---

* *thyrotoxic periodic paralysis (TPP)*

This would be a classic case. Seventy-five percent of TPP cases are in Asians, more than 80% have their onset in the third or fourth decade of life, and most of the victims are male.

These features help distinguish TPP from primary hypokalemic periodic paralysis. However, both conditions are similar in that (1) meals high in carbohydrate or sodium may provoke attacks, (2) exposure to cold or rest after exertion can precipitate attacks, (3) attacks may last minutes to days, and (4) both have decreased serum potassium levels during generalized attacks.

All cases of thyrotoxic periodic paralysis have been cured with the correction of the hyperthyroid state.

In 1943 an epidemic condition clinically resembling periodic paralysis was seen in China when massive contamination of table salt by barium chloride occurred.[4]

(1) Am J Med. **30**: 327-333 (1961). Periodic paralysis and thyroid function. Source of most of the above statistics. TPP is McKusick 17040.
(2) Mayo Clin Proc. **56**: 504-512 (1981). Neurologic aspects of thyroid dysfunction.
(3) Arch Intern Med. **148**: 708 only (1988). TPP in a Hispanic man.
(4) Neuromuscular Manifestations of Systemic Disease. RB Layzer. Philadelphia: FA Davis (1985). pp 54-57. Part of a section on barium poisoning.

---

* *patient is receiving L-dopa therapy for parkinsonism*[1,2]

L-dopa is a neutral amino acid that is transported across the blood-brain barrier by the "neutral amino acid transport system." Saturating the system with amino acids derived from dietary proteins can decrease the amount of L-dopa that reaches the brain, and is thought to be responsible for the "on-off" phenomenon seen in some parkinsonian patients taking L-dopa.[1]

Similarly, the anti-hypertensive alpha methyldopa (also known as Aldomet) administered with a high-protein meal is likely to be less effective in lowering blood pressure than if co-administered with a high carbohydrate meal.[1]

(1) Ann Intern Med. **105**: 82-95 (1986). Review of the blood-brain barrier. See EN-001.
(2) Arch Neurol. **44**: 1003-1005, 1006-1009 (1987). Diet and parkinsonism; two articles.

Diet DI-004

Pellagra,
despite a healthy diet

Diet DI-005

In a woman,
severe headaches after eating meat

Diet DI-006

Paper pica

* *carcinoid syndrome,*[1] *Hartnup disease,*[1] *isoniazid therapy*[2]

Pellagra results from niacin deficiency ("niacin" is generic for both nicotinic acid and nicotinamide). Because niacin is made from tryptophan in vivo, pellagra may result from a deficiency of either niacin or tryptophan. These deficiencies are not always dietary.

In the carcinoid syndrome up to 60% of tryptophan is catabolized to serotonin in what is normally a minor (1%) metabolic pathway. In Hartnup disease, tryptophan and other amino acids are poorly absorbed from both the gut and the renal tubule.[1] Other causes of malabsorption may also lead to pellagra.[3] Isoniazid blocks the conversion of tryptophan to niacin,[2] as does estrogen.[4] Niacin requirements are increased by thyrotoxicosis and by prolonged infections (for example, tuberculosis).[1]

When due to dietary deficiency, the manifestations of pellagra are always complicated by other deficiencies. Classically, however, the signs of pellagra are described as the three D's: diarrhea, dementia, and dermatitis.[1] Less than 25% of pellagrins will have the full triad.[5,6] Some add a fourth D: death.

(1) Cecil Textbook of Medicine. 16th ed. JB Wyngaarden & LH Smith Jr (eds). Philadelphia: Saunders (1982) p 1368.
(2) J Neurol Neurosurg Psych. **48**:628-634 (1985). Pellagra in 8% of TB patients on INH autopsied.
(3) Gastroenterology. **82**:948-952 (1982). Crohn disease, for example.
(4) Br J Nutr. **51**:219-224 (1984). May explain the 2:1 female:male ratio in pellagra.
(5) Johns Hopkins Med J. **140**:295-309 (1977). 18 patients and literature review.
(6) J Neurol Neurosurg Psych. **44**:209-215 (1981). Pellagra in 20 of 74 chronic alcoholics autopsied.
(–) Brain. **111**:829-842 (1988). Clinical spectrum of alcoholic pellagra encephalopathy.

---

* *ornithine transcarbamylase (OTC) deficiency* *(McKusick 31125)*

OTC, a hepatic enzyme of the urea cycle, catalyzes the formation of citrulline from carbamyl phosphate and ornithine. Deficiency of OTC, an X-linked trait, results in hyperammonemia.[1] Affected males have no OTC activity and die in the neonatal period.[2] In [heterozygous] females, however, random inactivation of affected X chromosomes (the Lyon phenomenon) results in some hepatocytes with normal OTC activity. Owing to this mosaicism, symptoms in females are variable, ranging from none to severe mental and physical retardation.[1]

Formerly thought to appear by the end of the first decade of life or not at all, onset of severe symptoms in the late 30s was recently reported in two women.[1] In each case, superimposed liver disease (due to alcohol and cytomegalovirus, respectively) probably contributed to adult unmasking of OTC deficiency. One also had a lifelong history of headaches precipitated by eating meat, as has been reported several times in asymptomatic women with OTC deficiency. These headaches may be labelled "migraine" because they are accompanied by nausea, vomiting, and, occasionally, by neurologic signs. Catabolic stress (such as surgery) or high protein/high nitrogen meals can precipitate the headaches.[1,3] Thus, an aversion to high protein meals may develop early in life.[1,4]

(1) Ann Intern Med. **106**:556-558 (1987). Nice discussion; case reports of two women.
(2) Exceptions: [a] New Engl J Med. **315**:744-747 (1986). [b] New Engl J Med. **319**:999-1003 (1988).
(3) Interestingly, gout attacks are similarly provoked. [Scientific American Medicine. 15:IX:4 (5/86).]
(4) Carriers of other urea cycle enzyme defects may have similar headaches. [The Metabolic Basis of Inherited Disease. 5th ed. JB Stanbury et al (eds). New York: McGraw-Hill (1983). p 414.]

---

* *may cause mercury poisoning*

In the case reported,[1] a 46-year-old woman with iron deficiency anemia was found to have the highest hair mercury content in Manitoba. For 12 years she had had an intense craving for paper, recently satisfied by consuming a Kleenex box and a cigarette package daily, and, before that, by eating an entire paperback book each day. Her staples were analyzed for mercury content: Kleenex box – 83 ppb; cigarette package – 108 ppb; pages of a paperback book – 341 ppb. (Parts per billion are equivalent to micrograms per kilogram of body weight.) After a week of iron replacement her pica resolved; within several months her hair mercury levels normalized.

Mercury is used as an antifungal agent in the pulp and paper industry.[1] Previously, it was used to cure felt, which resulted in many hatters becoming poisoned by mercury, hence the character of the Mad Hatter in *Alice's Adventures in Wonderland.*[2] Today, over 50 occupations involve potential exposure to mercury; dentists, photographers, histology technicians, wood preservative workers, and paper pulp workers are at risk.[3]

Mercury's toxicity depends on both its chemical state (elemental, organic, inorganic salt) and its route of entry (inhalation *vs* ingestion). Clinical presentations range from chronic nonspecific psychological effects to acute cardiovascular collapse.[3]

(1) New Engl J Med. **306**:1056-1057 (1982). Letter.
(2) The Annotated Alice. L Carroll. Annotated by M Gardner. New York: Bramhall (1960). p 90.
(3) Goldfrank's Toxicologic Emergencies. 3rd ed. L Goldfrank et al (eds). Norwalk, CT: Appleton-Century-Crofts (1986). pp 640-650.
(–) FDA Drug Bull. **13(1)**:5-6 (1983). Death after merthiolate irrigation of a child's ear. (Hamlet!)
(–) Lancet. **II**:1095, 1335 (1987). Paper pica mimicking porphyria.

Diet DI-007

Acquired trait of passing red urine
after eating beets

Diet DI-008

Return in later life of
cravings or aversions experienced in pregnancy

Ear EA-001

Diagonal ear lobe crease

(beeturia)

* *iron deficiency*[1]

Beet pigment (betacyanin) is renally excreted, and colors acidic urine pink to deep red. Fourteen percent of normal persons develop visible beeturia after ingesting beets, *perhaps* on a genetic basis (McKusick 10960).

However, when 100 g of small beets ("much more than anyone would eat from free choice") were fed to patients with untreated iron deficiency anemia,[1] 80% developed beeturia. Of 15 similar patients who had already received iron, only one developed beeturia, suggesting that betacyanin absorption, and hence beeturia, occurs at times of "iron hunger." Consistent with this was the 46% incidence of beeturia in pernicious anemia patients (augmented iron absorption occurs in this disease during vitamin B_{12} treatment) and the 33% incidence in non-anemic patients with both malabsorption and biopsy-proven jejunal atrophy[1] (the jejunum plays an important role in iron absorption[2]).

It has been suggested that iron and betacyanin compete for an intestinal acceptor substance, with iron the preferred ligand. Because beeturia can appear and disappear in normals, at least some of the "baseline" 14% incidence may be due to the fluctuating nature of iron absorption in normal people.[1]

Other effects of vegetables on the sensorium include the olfactory repercussions of asparagus metabolites in urine (McKusick 10840) and the way artichokes make water taste sweet to some individuals (McKusick 10832).

(1) Br Med J. **2**: 971-973 (1963). Study from Scotland.
(2) Annu Rev Med. **34**: 55-68 (1983). Review of iron absorption.

---

* *cancer*[1]

This association emerged from interviews of 1237 hospital patients; 850 were attending a radiotherapy and oncology center and the rest were inpatients "with no overt tumor." Twenty-four women (22 of whom had a tumor) were found who in later life had the same craving(s) or aversion(s) they had had in pregnancy, or the opposite feeling for the same substance; 85% of cases involved edible substances, and most were aversions, usually associated temporally with the development or treatment of the tumor.[1]

Although uncontrolled, the study above adds a third class of appetite perversions to the well-known, but pathogenetically obscure, pica of iron deficiency[2,3,4] and cissa of pregnancy.[2,5] Patients with pica will never volunteer information about their cravings; they are ashamed of it and must be asked directly.[3,6] Some forms are dangerous and must be detected (for example, paper pica, card DI-006),[7] but even the casual ice-chewer may welcome reassurance that she (less frequently, he) is not crazy.

(1) Lancet. **II**: 907-908 (1980). Study is re-hashed in: Clin Radiol. **33**: 471-475 (1982).
(2) Pica (from the Latin for "magpie") is "a depraved or perverted appetite; a hunger for substances unfit as food." Cissa is "a craving for unusual or unwholesome articles of food; the unnatural longings of pregnancy." [Stedman's Medical Dictionary]
(3) JAMA. **235**: 2765 only (1976). Up to 50% of patients with iron deficiency anemia have pica.
(4) Am J Med. **73**: 931-932 (1982). A cancer patient with pica secondary to iron deficiency.
(5) "Cravings, aversions and pica of pregnancy." WH Trethowan & G Dickens. In: Modern Perspectives in Psycho-Obstetrics. JG Howells (ed). Edinburgh: Oliver & Boyd (1972). pp 251-268.
(6) Etched in memory is the smile of the young anemic woman asked "How much ice do you eat?" In the Book of Prognostics, Hippocrates notes the great impact of explaining patients' "omissions."
(7) Am Fam Physician. **33(5)**: 181-185 (1986). Also says to ask criminals about blood-sucking.

---

* *coronary artery disease (CAD)*[1,2]

After more than 30 studies the reliability of this sign remains controversial.[1,2] Key issues in the debate are the population to which the sign is applied and the disputed age-independence of ear lobe creases.

Thus, attempts to increase the sign's predictive value have been made (but not validated). These suggestions often incorporate coexistent physical findings, for example:

- hair in the ear canal;[3]
- mesomorphic body build plus premature baldness;[4]
- "atherosclerotic facies," which is said to include ear lobe creases[5] and be similar to, but distinct from, the recently described "smoker's face."[5,6]

Ear lobe creases are part of the Beckwith and the SPEL syndromes[7] and may be associated with other disorders.[1,2] Apparently the Roman emperor Hadrian (AD 76-138) had coronary artery disease, type A behavior, and bilateral ear lobe creases.[8]

(1) Am J Med. **75**: 1024-1032 (1983). Literature review and study of 1000 patients. Here, the sign was 60% sensitive and 65% selective for CAD, hence more reliable than "traditional" risk factors.
(2) Arch Intern Med. **147**: 65-66 (1987). Found no independent correlation with CAD.
(3) New Engl J Med. **311**: 1317-1318 (1984). Letter describing a study of 63 patients.
(4) Essentials of Cardiac Diagnosis. J Abrams. Philadelphia: Lea & Febiger (1987). p 187.
(5) TA Traill, MRCP. Johns Hopkins Hospital. November 1988.
(6) Br Med J. **291**: 1755, 1760-1762 (1985). Smoker's face.
(7) Beckwith is McKusick 13065; SPEL is McKusick 18635; ear lobe creases are McKusick 12895.
(8) West J Med. **132**: 87-91 (1980). Cited by reference 1.

Ear EA-002

Acute vertigo when patient presses on tragus

Ear EA-003

Ear pain

Ear EA-004

Patient intermittently hears a high-pitched buzzing, coming from one to two meters above his head

(Hennebert symptom)

* *perilymphatic fistula*

Perilymphatic fistulae are abnormal openings in the round and/or oval windows that allow communication between the perilymph (the fluid surrounding the membranous labyrinth) and the middle ear space. They occur at any age and are difficult to diagnose preoperatively; patients present with an "amazing array" of signs and symptoms, and conclusive preoperative tests do not exist.[1] Predisposing factors include prior otologic surgery, trauma, exertion/straining, and upper respiratory infections. Roughly a third of cases are idiopathic or due to congenital malformations.[1]

Hearing loss (involving any frequency), vestibular symptoms (of any kind), tinnitus, and sensations of aural fullness may occur with any chronicity or may not occur at all. Surgery eliminates or improves symptoms in 90% of patients. Vertigo induced by straining (for example, during defecation) or by exertion (even as little as vacuuming) is a classic symptom. Pressing on the tragus causes vertigo by inducing a change in air pressure in the external ear canal: The perilymphatic fistula allows transmission of this pressure change to the endolymphatic space, wherein lie components of the vestibular apparatus.[1]

The Hennebert sign is eye deviation provoked by pneumatic otoscopy.[1]

(1) Laryngoscope. **94**: 37-49 (1986). 91 patients with proven PLFs.
(–) Ann Otol Rhinol Laryngol. **88**: 153-159 (1979). Perilymphatic fistulae with vertigo and Hennebert sign, but without hearing loss.
(–) Ann Otol Rhinol Laryngol. **97**: 105-108 (1988). Seeks indications for surgical exploration.

(otalgia)

* *not necessarily due to otic pathology*

Pain in the ear can be referred from any structure in proximity to cranial nerves V, IX, X, or cervical nerves C1, C2, C3:

- dental or oral disease (nerve V)
- tongue or tonsils (nerve IX)
- pharynx
- larynx (nerve X)
- esophagus
- thyroid
- sinuses
- temporomandibular joint
- lung or bronchus
- elongation of the styloid process or ossification of stylohyoid ligament
- various neuralgias
- cervical spine lesions
- angina pectoris
- thoracic aneurysm
- innominate artery aneurysm
- chilblains

Eye Ear Nose Throat Monthly. **46**: 587-588 (1967). Differential diagnosis of referred otalgia.
Otolaryngology. M Paparella & D Shumrick. Philadelphia: Saunders (1980). pp 1354-1357.

---

* *patient is in a radar beam*[1,2]

"Hear" is the wrong word; it appears the human central nervous system is stimulated directly: At the threshold of radar "hearing," the average sound pressure of the radar wave is roughly three orders of magnitude below the threshold pressure for conventional hearing.[1] Radars operating at 1, 3, and 10 gigahertz have been heard.

The sound is "something like that of a bee buzzing on a window, but with, perhaps, more high frequencies." A window screen with a hole cut in it (to localize the radar beam) showed that "the only part of the body which allowed the observer to hear the radar was a place on the head above the forehead.... Placing the fingers in the ears in reasonable ambient noise did not seem greatly to affect the threshold value at which the radar [was] heard."

A similar phenomenon may occur with electromagnetic waves from meteors and aurorae.[1] Equally intriguing is that muscular activity in humans can be induced by non-invasive magnetic stimulation of the motor cortex.[3] Human ears *emit* sounds.[4,5]

(1) NY State J Med. **67**: 2992-2997 (1967). Sensation of hearing in electromagnetic fields.
(2) Incredible Life: A Handbook of Biological Mysteries. WR Corliss. Glen Arm, MD: The Sourcebook Project (1981). p 110. Refers to the article above.
(3) Lancet. **I**: 1106-1107 (1985). Non-invasive magnetic stimulation of the motor cortex.
(4) Science News. **128**: 328 only (1985). Why almost 50% of people do this, no one knows.
(5) Science News. **129**: 122 only (1986). Elephants emit low frequency sounds from their foreheads.
(–) Aerosp Med. **35**: 834-839 (1964). Alternating electric fields can be heard with the ears.
(–) Other hazards of electromagnetism appear on card HE-002.

Ear EA-005

Pneumonia and bullous myringitis

Ear EA-006

Calcification of the pinna

Ear EA-007

Inflammation of the external ear,
sparing the lobe

* Mycoplasma pneumoniae *pneumonia*

This community-acquired pneumonia usually occurs in healthy young adults (the highest risk is from ages 5 to 20).[1] Two thirds of patients will have nonspecific ear complaints[2] and 10% to 15% will have frank myringitis.[1,3] Bullous myringitis, which develops less often, appears as large hemorrhagic bullae on the tympanic membrane, from which *M. pneumoniae* may be isolated. The bullae heal without scarring.[3]

Onset of disease is insidious. Constitutional symptoms such as fever, malaise, and headache are usually present 2 to 4 days before the disease localizes.[1] Cough, typically nonproductive, becomes a prominent manifestation; its absence makes the diagnosis unlikely.[1] Because of the delayed flowering of pulmonary findings, patients may at first appear much more ill than physical findings suggest.[3] Hospitalization is generally not required.[1]

The leukocyte count is normal 85% of the time. On the chest film, infiltrates may be segmental, lobar, or diffusely reticulonodular. Cold agglutinins develop in one half of patients, but will occur more frequently in severely ill patients.[3]

(1) Principles and Practice of Infectious Diseases. 2nd ed. GL Mandell et al (eds). New York: Wiley (1985). pp 1065-1076.
(2) Am J Med. **58**: 229-242 (1975). Protean manifestations of this disease.
(3) Medical Microbiology and Infectious Diseases. A Braude. Phila.: Saunders (1981). pp 925-929.

---

* *Endocrinopathies: Addison disease, diabetes mellitus, acromegaly, others*
* *Chondropathies: alkaptonuria, relapsing polychondritis, others*
* *Trauma: frostbite, mechanical trauma, radiotherapy*
* *Systemic calcium derangements: hyperparathyroidism, sarcoidosis, others*
* *Other: apparently normal persons, scleroderma, others!*

Over 140 cases and almost 30 causes of auricular calcification had been reported through 1985.[1,2,3] In 128 cases reviewed in 1964, the most common causes were frostbite (30 cases), ear trauma/mechanical factors (17), Addison disease (14), acromegaly (5), alkaptonuria (4), diabetes mellitus (4), relapsing polychondritis (3), and "idiopathic" (43).[2]

The condition may not be uncommon: 11 of 300 consecutive inpatients (in Chicago) had auricular calcification on physical examination confirmed by x-ray(!), and in 12 patients with diseases predisposing to heterotopic calcification, x-rays disclosed another three cases.[2] Inexplicably, no cases have been reported in women.[4] Calcification may involve the entire auricle, leaving it stiff and rigid, or only a portion of it. In cases that progress to ossification, extension of the bony deposits into the ear canal may lead to external otalgia that is aggravated by sleeping in the lateral decubitus position.[1]

(1) Laryngoscope. **95**: 566-576 (1985). Review of auricular calcification. See also card EA-008.
(2) Arch Intern Med. **113**: 23-27 (1964). Another review, with 114 prior and 14 new cases.
(3) Causes not covered in references 1 and 2 are: prolactinoma [Med Clin (Barcelona). **85**: 557-558 (1985).] and diastrophic dwarfism [New Engl J Med. **270**: 319 only (1964).].
(4) J Clin Endocrinol Metab. **55**: 354-357 (1983). Three cases in men with hypopituitarism.

---

* *relapsing polychondritis (RP)*[1]

When the external ear becomes inflamed, it can be difficult to distinguish infectious from noninfectious causes such as relapsing polychondritis. Because the lobule is the only part of the ear that lacks cartilage, it is not involved by RP.

Although clinical criteria have been suggested to establish a diagnosis of RP, recurrent chondritis of both external ears is "virtually pathognomonic" of the disease. These repeated bouts of chondritis can result in cauliflower ear or calcification of the pinna (card EA-006).

Relapsing polychondritis may also involve the cardiovascular system and the respiratory passages, sometimes fatally. Biopsy of tracheal or bronchial cartilage is ill-advised when RP is suspected, as collapse and severe airway obstruction can occur. Likewise, collapse of cartilage in the nasal bridge, resulting in a saddle-nose deformity, may also be part of the illness.

(1) New Engl J Med. **312**: 1695-1703 (1985). CPC on progressive saddle-nose deformity.
(–) Ann Intern Med. **109**: 163-164 (1988). Color illustration.

Ear EA-008

Bony growths in external ear canal

Ear EA-009

Hypesthesia of the posterior wall
of the external auditory canal

Ear EA-010

Punctate red opacifications detected
by transillumination of the ear lobe

(meatal exostoses)

* *history of cold-water swimming*

These exostoses are new growths of bone arising from the osseous portion of the external auditory canal (EAC). When present, they are usually multiple and bilateral, and "appear as discrete, round, ovoid, or elongated excrescences with small, almost pedunculated bases, or as diffuse bulges of ivory-like bone."[1] Chronic irritation of the EAC (for example, from infection, eczema, or trauma) causes exostoses,[2] but their most common cause is swimming in cold water.[1] The prevalence of ear exostoses in a male English population was 0.7%, all occurring in individuals giving a history of regular swimming.[3]

Cold water is a strong irritant to the EAC: A 15-second irrigation of the skin of the EAC with 40°C water produces erythema lasting 1 minute; using 15°C water, however, yields 45 minutes of erythema.[2] Exostoses remain asymptomatic unless they cause retention of water or debris.[1]

In contrast to exostoses, osteomas are relatively rare, usually single, bony growths of the EAC. They have a more pedunculated base and the appearance of a foreign body or cyst. Removal is advised because their continued growth eventually occludes the canal.[3,4] Calcification of the pinna (card EA-006) can, in advanced cases, cause calcification of the EAC as well.[5]

(1) Pathology of the Ear. HF Schuknecht. Cambridge, MA: Harvard (1974). p 383.
(2) Otolaryngology. M Paparella & D Shumrick. Philadelphia: Saunders (1980). pp 1360-1361.
(3) J Laryngol Otol. **65**: 704-714 (1951). A sparkling, intellectual study of the topic.
(4) Laryngoscope. **68**: 1667-1673 (1958). Sketch illustrations of osteoma and exostosis.
(5) Laryngoscope. **95**: 566-576 (1985). Has an incorrect reference to an ear exostosis article.

(Hitselberger sign)

* *early sign of acoustic neuroma*

The internal auditory canal (IAC) is the home to the facial, cochlear, and vestibular nerves. It is the last of these that gives rise to acoustic neuromas. Because sensory nerves are more susceptible to pressure than are motor nerves, acoustic neuromas cause hearing loss, tinnitus, and dysequilibrium (though usually not frank vertigo) before facial weakness.[1]

Branches of the facial nerve do, however, serve two sensory functions: (1) The chorda tympani supplies taste to the anterior two thirds of the tongue, and (2) minute nerve branches originating in the IAC vestigially innervate the skin of the posterior wall of the external auditory canal (EAC). Compression of these nerve branches by a growing acoustic neuroma produces the Hitselberger sign.[1]

Complete anesthesia of the EAC's posterior wall is never produced because of the cutaneous sensory overlap between the trigeminal nerve superiorly and the cervical nerves inferiorly. Hitselberger originally observed that, in patients later shown to have acoustic neuroma, cold water caloric testing elicited considerably less pain on the side ipsilateral to the tumor than on the side contralateral to it. He later used a "right angle hook" to elicit the sign, which is claimed as 95% sensitive for detecting facial nerve involvement.[1]

Less than 10% of acoustic neuromas are bilateral (but see card FA-003).

(1) Am Surg. **32**: 741-743 (1966). Original description.
(–) Neurology. **33**: 211-221 (1983). Atypical features of acoustic neuroma.
(–) Laryngoscope. **88**: 1893-1903 (1978). Symptoms and signs in 225 acoustic neuroma patients.

---

* *subacute bacterial endocarditis (SBE)*[1a]

Eponymously known as "Libman spots," an embolic or vasculitic cause for them seems plausible. The frequency of this sign is not stated.

Interestingly, another ear lobe sign of SBE exists: the presence of histiocytes (that is, macrophages) in blood expressed from the lobule. Presumably the result of cell filtering by the lobule's vasculature, finding large numbers of such cells is highly suggestive of SBE if a few other conditions can be excluded.[2]

Although it almost seems a joke of nature that ear lobes can serve as diagnostic aids, recall cards EA-001 and EA-007 and consider the following:

- large ear lobes "occur characteristically in some of the mucopolysaccharidoses;"[3]
- pulsatile ear lobes are "always due to venous rather than arterial pulsation;"[4]
- nodules in the ear lobes may be associated with Peyronie disease;[5]
- anterior-pointing ear lobes are part of the facies of Noonan syndrome;[6]
- puffy, enlarged ear lobes are very common in lepromatous leprosy;[1b]
- bluish-red inflammation of a child's ear lobe signals Lyme disease.[7]

(1) Clinical Diagnostic Pearls. JC Birnholz & PE Michelson. Flushing, NY: Medical Examination (1971). [a] p 15; [b] p 61; card HD-301 explains why.
(2) J Lab Clin Med. **48**: 827-845 (1956). A detailed review of ear lobe histiocytes.
(3) Facial Features of Neurologic Syndromes. PR Dyken & MD Miller. St. Louis: Mosby (1980). p 81.
(4) Clinical Cardiology. 2nd ed. M Sokolow & MB McIlroy. Los Altos, CA: Lange (1979). p 43.
(5) Lecture Notes on Urology. 3rd ed. J Blandy. Oxford: Blackwell (1982). p 263.
(6) TA Traill, MRCP. Johns Hopkins Hospital Medical Grand Rounds, 1 May 1982.
(7) Ann NY Acad Sci. **539**: 4-15 (1988). Cutaneous manifestations of Lyme disease.

Endocrine EN-001

Diabetic with classic symptoms of hypoglycemia,
but with a normal serum glucose level

Extremities EX-001

Excruciating limb pain
during hot weather or fevers

Extremities EX-002

Warmth, congestion, redness, and burning pain
in a limb when it is exposed to heat

** brain glucopenia*

Glucose reaches the brain via a glucose transport system at the blood-brain barrier. In patients with poorly controlled diabetes, chronically elevated serum glucose levels (over 300 mg/dL) cause down-regulation of this transport system. Thus, when insulin therapy achieves rapid control of serum glucose in these patients, brain glucopenia may result because a "normal" serum glucose level is too low to drive sufficient glucose through the transport system and into the brain.[1]

Similarly, chronic hypoglycemia causes an up-regulation of the transport system, which may explain why some patients with insulinoma do not have symptoms of brain glucopenia despite serum glucose concentrations of less than 50 mg/dL.[1]

Seizures or aspirin intoxication can raise the brain's glucose demands. Thus, they may cause brain glycopenia in the presence of normal or even elevated levels of serum glucose.[1]

(1) Ann Intern Med. **105**: 82-95 (1986). Review of the blood-brain barrier. See DI-003 also.
(–) Mayo Clin Proc. **60**: 844-850 (1985). Review of hypoglycemia.
(–) New Engl J Med. **318**: 1523-1532 (1988). CPC on hypoglycemia.
(–) New Engl J Med. **318**: 1487-1492 (1988). Altered threshold for hypoglycemic symptoms in diabetics.

** Fabry disease*

Eighty to ninety percent of males with this X-linked lipid storage disorder experience a painful neuropathy, usually beginning in childhood or adolescence. Two kinds of pain have been described: (1) A nagging, constant burning or tingling in the hands and feet (acroparesthesias), and (2) attacks of severe pain lasting hours or days (Fabry crises) that are triggered by fever, a warm environment, exercise, fatigue, emotional stress, or any rapid change in temperature and humidity.[1] (Note the similarities to the Uhthoff phenomenon in multiple sclerosis – card EY-001.)

Acroparesthesias may worsen in the afternoon[1] (which is when a diurnal increase in body temperature normally occurs[2]). Female carriers, who may suffer such multiple sclerosis-like symptoms as episodic vertigo, visual loss, dysarthria, and hemiparesis, have noted acroparesthesias after running two miles.[3]

Despite the histologic and electrical abnormalities of these patients' nerves,[1] clinical neurologic examination is often negative,[3] leading to such misdiagnoses as rheumatic fever, erythromelalgia (see card EX-002), collagen vascular disease, or neurosis.[1]

Fabry patients do poorly in the heat for another reason: anhidrosis, possibly caused by sweat gland atrophy or autonomic neuropathy.[1,3] The skin may turn beet red on exposure to heat,[3] and heat stroke during military training is frequent.[4]

(1) The Metabolic Basis of Inherited Disease. 5th ed. JB Stanbury et al (eds). New York: McGraw-Hill (1983). pp 906-944. Review of Fabry disease.
(2) Rev Infect Dis. **7**: 692-699 (1985). Clinically benign fevers of unknown origin.
(3) New Engl J Med. **310**: 106-114 (1984). CPC, with extensive discussion of pain in Fabry disease.
(4) Harrison's Principles of Internal Medicine. 11th ed. E Braunwald et al (eds). New York: McGraw-Hill (1987). p 1669.

** erythromelalgia*

Erythromelalgia most often affects the lower limbs or all four limbs; in 50% of patients with affected lower limbs, the distress is confined to the soles of the feet. Attacks usually last a few hours (range, minutes to 2 days), during which the pain is "moderately severe."[1] Unlike the acral pains of Fabry disease (card EX-201), which are precipitated to a greater extent by a rise in body temperature than they are by raising the external temperature of a limb,[2] erythromelalgic paroxysms are usually prompted by heating of, or by prolonged dependence of, a susceptible extremity.[1] Thus, walking, standing, exercising, sleeping under covers, wearing shoes/gloves, or placing the limb near a heater are classic provocations. The frequency and/or severity of attacks may increase in summer.[1]

Relief is obtained by elevating or cooling the affected limb(s), *eg*, by walking on a cold floor. Some patients routinely sleep with their feet outside the covers.[1,3] A single low dose of aspirin may relieve pain for 2 to 4 days, a response that is almost diagnostic.[4]

Erythromelalgia is sometimes associated with chronic myeloproliferative disorders (especially polycythemia vera and primary thrombocythemia), and may develop years before them.[4] Although its cause is unknown, fascinating reports on the role of platelets have recently appeared.[5]

(1) Circulation. **29**: 136-141 (1964). 51 cases of "erythermalgia."
(2) Neurology. **32**: 498-502 (1982). Autonomic dysfunction in Fabry disease.
(3) Hippocrates thought this a bad prognostic sign in illness, "for it indicates aberration of intellect." [The Complete Works of Hippocrates. F Adams (transl). Book of Prognostics, paragraph 3.]
(4) Arch Intern Med. **149**: 105-109 (1989). Erythromelalgia and myeloproliferative disorders.
(5) Ann Intern Med. **102**: 466-471; **103**: 473 only (1985). Erythromelalgia and platelets.

Extremities - Hands and Feet EX-201

High arches

Extremities - Hands and Feet EX-202

In a woman,
big toe widely separated from the rest of the toes

Extremities - Hands and Feet EX-203

Spontaneous amputation of little toe

(pes cavus)

* *familial degenerative neurologic disease (Charcot-Marie-Tooth disease, Freidreich ataxia, hereditary spastic paraplegia, Roussy-Lévy syndrome, myelodysplasia, spina bifida, Refsum disease)*
* *relatives of people afflicted as above*
* *isolated familial cases without family history of neurologic disease*
* *pes cavus and lymphedema syndrome*

Of 77 patients seen in a pes cavus clinic, one third had Charcot-Marie-Tooth disease, one third had other neurologic disease (myelodysplasia, polio, and Freidreich ataxia the most common), and one third had idiopathic pes cavus. In this final third, one half had a family history of pes cavus.[2]

Patients with the Marfan syndrome may have pes cavus, but flat feet (pes planus) are "much more common."[3]

(1) Handbook of Clinical Neurology. **21**: 263-269 (1975). The differential listed above.
(2) Br Med J. **2**: 659-661 (1963). Pes cavus clinic.
(3) Heritable Disorders of Connective Tissue. 4th ed. VA McKusick. St. Louis: Mosby (1972). p 82.

---

* *prostitution*[1]

According to the Italian physician Cesare Lombroso at the 1886 International Congress on Criminal Anthropology, this prehensile type of foot is an atavistic anomaly. This "fact" was consistent with his famous (but now defunct) theory that the physiognomy of criminals resembled that of apes (low forehead, long arms, and so forth).

We also have Lombroso to thank for the idea that almost "every born criminal is an epileptic."

(1) The Mismeasure of Man. SJ Gould. New York: Norton (1981). pp 123-134.
(–) In a serious vein, this finding is the Goldstein sign of Down syndrome [Atlas of Pediatric Physical Diagnosis. BJ Zitelli & HW Davis. St. Louis: Mosby (1987). p 1.7]. Toe spacing may be inherited as an irregular autosomal dominant trait (McKusick 18923).
(–) The actual point of this card, lost on many early readers, is that the sometimes preposterous seeming associations found on other cards may someday prove to be just that, despite their "authoritative" documentation.

---

* *ainhum*[1] *(dactylosis spontanea)*

The name "ainhum" means "to saw or cut" in the Nago dialect.[2] Bloodless autoamputation is the result of a "progressive fibrotic groove or fissure formation encircling one or more toes,"[1] most often the little toe. Adults of the darker-skinned races living in the tropics or subtropics are primarily afflicted, but cases have been seen both in black and white Americans.[2,3,4] There are no known systemic abnormalities associated with this curious disorder, whose total course runs months to years.

Three possible causes of ainhum have been proposed:[5] (1) Overproduction of fibrous tissue in response to injury and infection.[4] This would account for the role that going barefoot seems to play, and also link ainhum with keloids; (2) Absence of the [arterial] plantar arch, resulting in diminished blood supply to the little toe;[6] and (3) A toxic cause, possibly of plant origin.

(1) NY State J Med. **81**: 1779-1781 (1981). Short review; illustrated.
(2) Arch Dermatol Syphilol. **36**: 1058-1063 (1937). Six cases in New York City blacks.
(3) JAMA. **246**: 1591-1592 (1981). Case in an American black man.
(4) J Bone Joint Surg (British). **47B**: 43-51, 52-55 (1965). Older reviews.
(5) Manson's Tropical Diseases. 19th ed. PEC Manson-Bahr & DR Ball. London: Ballière Tindall (1987). pp 1130-1132.
(6) Lancet. **II**: 396-397 (1981). Normally, the plantar arch arises from the posterior tibial artery and, with branches of the dorsalis pedis artery, co-supplies the toes.
(–) "Ainhum has attracted far more attention than its importance merits" [Int J Dermatol. **15**: 348-350 (1976).]. It may also be familial (McKusick 10340).
(–) The sensation of a band around the toe may be an early symptom of multiple sclerosis. [McAlpine's Multiple Sclerosis. WB Matthews et al. Edinburgh: Churchill Livingstone (1985). p 103.]

Extremities - Hands and Feet

EX-204

Bullae on a woman's toes

Extremities - Hands and Feet

EX-205

Fingertip skin does not become wrinkled after prolonged immersion in warm water

Extremities - Lower

EX-401

Venous stasis in a man

* *porphyria cutanea tarda (PCT)*

Abnormally high blood and tissue levels of uroporphyrin cause the mild to severe photosensitivity of PCT.[1] Open-toed shoes, predominantly worn by women, expose the toes to light. In PCT this results in skin fragility, marked by vesicles, bullae, skin shearing, and scars. Most patients do not associate sun exposure with the development of new skin lesions.[2,3]

PCT is the most common form of porphyria and usually appears in middle or late adult life (hence, "tarda"). Patients, who frequently have evidence of liver disease, are at increased risk for hepatoma. Alcohol, estrogens, and hepatic siderosis predispose to PCT.[1] Hereditary cases are less common than sporadic ones.[4] PCT can be successfully treated by phlebotomy.[1]

Epidemics of PCT-like disease may occur from chemical exposure, as in the case of the "Turkish monkey children."[5]

(1) The Metabolic Basis of Inherited Disease. 5th ed. JB Stanbury et al (eds). New York: McGraw-Hill (1983). pp 1301-1384. Thorough discussion of all six types of porphyria.
(2) Am J Med. **67**: 277-286 (1979). Clinical and lab features of PCT. Illustrations.
(3) Arch Dermatol. **119**: 84-87 (1983). Case of a male sandal wearer. Color illustraion.
(4) McKusick 17069 & 17610. Two forms of PCT.
(5) JAMA. **183**: 88-91 (1963). A devastating disease. Illustrated.
(–) The bullae of Weber-Cockayne syndrome, though localized to the hands and feet, are dependent not on light, but on temperature and friction (McKusick 13180).

---

* *peripheral sympathetic dysfunction in the limbs*

The phenomenon of fingertip wrinkling (which is assessed in a standardized manner by immersing the hands in 40°C tap water for 30 minutes) is thought to depend on two sets of factors: epidermal and deep-tissue.[1]

After immersion, the stratum corneum of the epidermis absorbs water and swells.[2] Provided the turgor of the deep tissues is sufficiently low, swelling of the epidermis will lead to wrinkling. When sympathetic tone is low or nil, however, blood vessels are dilated and tissue turgor is too great to allow wrinkling. (Edema may have the same effect.)[1]

Thus, the test is valuable because it is easy to apply and because, unlike most other bedside tests of sympathetic function, it reflects peripheral rather than cardiac sympathetic denervation.[1] Absence of the wrinkling response is seen in some patients with the neuropathy of diabetes mellitus or Guillain-Barré syndrome.[1] All patients with Fabry disease, a lipid storage disorder partly characterized by a generalized autonomic neuropathy (see card EX-001), appear to lack the wrinkling response as well.[3]

(1) Br Med J. **1**: 551-552 (1977). All about fingertip wrinkling.
(2) The water's pH, temperature, and salt content influence the degree of epidermal hydration. Only the palms and soles wrinkle because they lack sebaceous glands, sebum exerting a waterproofing effect. [reference 1]
(3) Neurology. **32**: 498-502 (1982). But by what age? The youngest tested was 16.
(–) Another subtle sign of sympathetic dysfunction would be an inability to develop "gooseflesh," since piloerection is similarly mediated [Medical Physiology. 14th ed. VB Mountcastle (ed). St. Louis: Mosby (1980). pp 897-899.]. But try developing a standardized stimulus for gooseflesh....
(–) Quicker-than-normal fingertip wrinkling is a sign of cystic fibrosis [Lancet. **II**: 108, 907 (1974).].

---

* *decreased marriage rates and, in those who are married, decreased number of children*

This association emerged when 80 consecutive men being treated at a skin clinic for severe venous stasis (of whom 67 had stasis ulcers) were compared with 80 age-matched controls. Several differences were found: The stasis group was heavier (by 8 kg), taller (by 3.3 cm), and slightly more obese than the controls. Men in the stasis group were or had been married less often (64% *vs* 93%), if married were less likely to have had children (69% *vs* 84%), and, if a father, had fewer children (1.28 *vs* 1.97).

Because men with the Klinefelter syndrome (XXY genotype) are tall, obese, and have a high prevalence of venous stasis and leg ulcers, the authors karyotyped 15 of the unmarried men with stasis ulcers and found two that were XXY (the incidence in the normal population is about 1 in 400).

Patients with Klinefelter syndrome also have moderate hypogonadism, due to partial gonadal failure. Thus, the authors postulate that relative androgen deficiency may predispose to venous stasis and ulceration, and that decreased marriage and fertility rates in men with severe venous stasis may be due to androgen deficiency as well. (Evidence against this hypothesis, however, is the measurement of normal salivary testosterone levels in 10 childless men from the stasis group.)

Lancet. **II**: 630 only (1982).

Extremities - Lower EX-402

Anterior bowing of the tibias

Extremities - Lower EX-403

Pain in the leg on sneezing

Extremities - Lower EX-404

Leg itches when patient stands up

(saber shins)

* *late congenital syphilis*[1]
* *rickets*
* *fractures, osteomyelitis, tumors*[2]

"Anterior bowing of the tibia is not sufficient of itself for the diagnosis of saber tibia.... The combination of bowing with thickening [of the bone] is essential to the full value of the sign."[1] The bowing occurs years after the initial infection and is caused by the deposition of new bone under the periosteum of the anterior aspect of the tibia. It may or may not be painless. (Card MO-003 distinguishes early from late congenital syphilis.)

Saber shins were found in about 4% of patients with congenital syphilis in the late 1960s and, although this was "formerly a frequent occurrence in congenital syphilis, it was probably the result of vitamin D deficiency, combined with syphilitic anterior periostitis, causing anterior rather than lateral bowing."[3]

(1) Modern Clinical Syphilology. 3rd ed. JH Stokes et al. Philadelphia: Saunders (1944). p 1130.
(2) Arch Dermatol. **102**: 78-83 (1970). Clinical signs of congenital lues.
(3) Arch Dermatol. **99**: 599-610 (1969). Ditto.
(–) The periostitis and/or osteitis of tertiary lues most frequently affects the tibia [Med Clin North Am. **48**: 667-697 (1964).].

(cough-pain sign)

* *superficial venous thrombosis*[1]
* *deep venous thrombosis*[2,3] *(?)*

This sign is a well-established indicator of superficial thrombophlebitis.[1] Another early description[4] noted its occurrence in 40% of "thrombophlebitis" cases, now apparently interpreted as meaning deep vein thrombosis.[2,3] In any case, "pain that occurs along the course of the thrombosed vein can be induced by sneezing or coughing. The pain disappears with digital compression of the vein proximal to the obstruction."[3]

Although the physical examination is notoriously unreliable in cases of deep vein thrombosis, the "earliest and perhaps most reliable indication of thrombophlebitis" is said to be a feeling of heaviness in the leg. This can precede the appearance of objective physical signs by 24 to 48 hours.[5]

(1) J Med Soc NJ. **47**: 164-166 (April 1950). Cough-pain sign in acute superficial thrombophlebitis.
(2) "Thrombophlebitis: early physical signs." N Shafer. Med Counterpoint. **4(2)**: 57-59 (Feb. 1972).
(3) DeGowin & DeGowin's Bedside Diagnostic Examination. 5th ed. RL DeGowin. New York: Macmillan (1987). p 442. Calls it the Louvel sign; cites reference 2.
(4) Arch mal Coeur. **45**: 630-632 (1952). Report of Louvel and Laubry; in French.
(5) JO Humphries, MD, quoted in: Clinical Diagnostic Pearls. JC Birnholz & PE Michelson. Flushing, NY: Medical Examination (1971). p 90.

---

* *autonomic dysfunction*

Orthostatic hypotension is, of course, a hallmark of autonomic dysfunction. Orthostatic leg itching has also been reported. Presumably, loss of normal neurovascular reflexes in the legs leads to increased filling of the venous capacitance bed when the patient stands. This, in turn, leads to stretching of the skin, hence itching.

Loss of vascular tone causes significant problems in patients with autonomic dysfunction including, in about 60%, supine hypertension. (That is, elevation of blood pressure only when the patient is supine – one should always check for postural changes in blood pressure before starting treatment for hypertension.)

About 20% of patients complain of nasal stuffiness (caused by dilated mucosal veins), which would seem to be only an inconvenience but can actually be life-threatening: Some patients will treat themselves with over-the-counter nasal decongestants containing sympathomimetics. Because of absent buffering reflexes as well as denervation hypersensitivity of alpha receptors throughout the body, this will greatly exacerbate any supine hypertension already present, and in some cases can lead to such catastrophes as intracerebral bleeds.

Am J Med. **70**: 1091-1096 (1981). The clinical spectrum of autonomic dysfunction.

Extremities - Lower EX-405

Cannot walk without pain in the legs,
but can run perfectly well

Extremities - Lower EX-406

Painless bilateral knee effusions
in an adolescent

Extremities - Lower EX-407

Large ring-shaped rash
on posterior thighs and buttocks,
in a traveller returning from Japan

** popliteal artery entrapment*

The problem is a congenital anomaly of either (1) the path of the popliteal artery as it passes near the gastrocnemius muscle, or (2) the insertion of the medial head of the gastrocnemius muscle. Whichever type of anomaly, with each plantar flexion the gastrocnemius intermittently occludes the popliteal artery, eventually leading to degeneration and thrombosis of the vessel. Loss of limb has been reported, as have post-stenotic aneurysms of the artery.[1]

Many patients are young male athletes, hardly the typical host for peripheral vascular disease. They describe progressive intermittent claudication of the foot and/or leg after walking only a few hundred yards. Early in the disease, prolonged leg exercise, such as running, fails to provoke symptoms, probably because the gastrocnemius must contract longer when walking than when running. Twenty-five percent of patients have bilateral pathology.[1]

Early diagnosis is important, but can be difficult. The popliteal and pedal pulses are usually diminished in the resting state or with special maneuvers (such as active plantar flexion), but normal subjects may exhibit this pulse reduction as well. The history helps differentiate this syndrome from posterior compartment syndromes. Bilateral arteriography is recommended. Treatment is surgical.[1]

(1) Am J Sports Med. **11**: 180-182 (1983). Case report and nice summary.
(–) Am J Sports Med. **11**: 177-179 (1983). Two cases.
(–) Emergency Medicine. **16(2)**: 65, 68 (1984). Rehash of reference 1.

(Clutton joints)

** late congenital syphilis*

This sign occurs in less than 5% of patients with late congenital syphilis. (Card MO-003 distinguishes early and late congenital syphilis.) It appears quietly near puberty, and may not be prevented by prior treatment with penicillin.[1]

First one knee, then the other, becomes swollen. "It is a painless synovitis with a doughy swelling of the joint; x-ray films show no bone involvement; the joint fluid shows a few lymphocytes but no [polys]."[2] Reference 2 states "there is no condition which mimics it," but tuberculous hydrarthrosis can closely simulate Clutton joints.[3]

(1) Arch Dermatol. **99**: 599-610 (1969). Signs of late congenital syphilis. Illustrated.
(2) Arch Dermatol. **102**: 78-83 (1970). Ditto.
(3) Modern Clinical Syphilology. 3rd ed. JH Stokes et al (eds). Philadelphia: Saunders (1944). pp 798-799, 808, 1131-1133. Illustrated.
(–) Syphilis: A Synopsis. US Dept. of Health, Education, & Welfare. Washington: US Government Printing Office (1968). pp 93, 94.

** poison ivy dermatitis (sort of)*[1]

The rash-provoking chemical in poison ivy is urushiol, a penta-decyl catechol.[2] The Japanese lacquer tree contains an urushiol-like substance, so when its lacquer is used to coat toilet seats, the above-mentioned rash may result. Other plant parts known to contain urushiol-like substances include the mango rind (leading to the unhappy "Florida grin") and cashew nut shells (much to the dismay of those who bought improperly shelled cashew nuts from a group of Pennsylvania Little Leaguers in 1982).[1,3] In poison ivy, poison oak, and poison sumac, urushiol flows in canals within the plants' leaves, stems, and roots; thus, the plant must be physically damaged before it can cause a rash.[1,2]

About half the population is sensitive to urushiol.[2] Avoidance can be difficult: Despite the Boy Scout admonition "leaves of three, let it be," poison ivy and poison oak exist in a "bewildering diversity" of forms.[1] Urushiol "sticks to anything," including skin, pets, and fomites. It can be depressingly persistent on skin, and, once on the hands, can be spread almost everywhere.[1]

Prompt washing with liberal quantities of water reduces the severity of dermatitis in all but the most sensitive people.[2] Reference 1 discusses many recent developments such as desensitization, immunization, and organo-clay.

(1) Hippocrates. **2 (4)**: 76-78, 80, 82 (1988). Amazingly practical article in a lay publication.
(2) J Invest Dermatol. **88 (3) Suppl.**: 7s-11s (1987). Source of many of reference 1's statements.
(3) J Am Acad Dermatol. **10**: 627-631 (1984). Dermatitis from cashew nuts.
(–) Loose association: A lavatory seat that feels cold only on one side is evidence for a localized loss of temperature sense, as seen in multiple sclerosis [McAlpine's Multiple Sclerosis. WB Matthews et al. Edinburgh: Churchill Livingstone (1985). p 103.].

Extremities - Upper EX-601

Hairy elbows

Eye EY-001

Diminished visual acuity
while taking a hot shower

Eye EY-002

Pulsating unilateral exophthalmos

* *hairy elbows syndrome*[1,2]

Technically known as familial hypertrichosis cubiti, this syndrome was first decribed in two Amish siblings. Other than short, but not dysplastic fingernails, no systemic ramifications could be found. In both cases, the hypertrichosis peaked at age 5.[1]

(1) J Med Genet. **7**: 158-160 (1970). More recent cases appear in: Arch Dermatol. **115**: 761 only; **116**: 19 only (1980).
(2) McKusick 13960.

(Uhthoff phenomenon[1])

* *multiple sclerosis (MS)*

Reduced nerve conductivity commonly occurs in MS patients after raising the body temperature; even a 0.5°C rise may worsen extant neurologic defects, cause reappearance of "healed" defects, or unmask subclinical disease. Exercise, fevers, warm weather, or hot showers or baths can cause not only diminished visual acuity, but many other possible neurologic signs.[2,3] Thus, a brisk walk may cause blurring of vision that resolves with rest, and a hot shower may lead to abrupt paraplegia.[4]

Because heat-induced neurologic signs usually resolve as body temperature normalizes, the "hot bath test" has been used to confirm suspected cases of MS.[5] The occasional permanence of heat-induced defects, however, makes such testing risky.[6] Other neurologic diseases demonstrate similar temperature-related phenomena, but do so less frequently and generally require a greater elevation of temperature.[7]

Cooling is often temporarily beneficial,[2] as in the patient whose visual acuity improved after drinking cold water.[8] However, it has also been reported to precipitate MS.[2]

(1) Uhthoff, in 1890, described temporary blurring of vision after exercise in MS patients (ref. 2).
(2) McAlpine's Multiple Sclerosis. WB Matthews et al. Edinburgh: Churchill Livingstone (1985). pp 90-91, 123, 221-223. 90% of MS patients notice a heat effect.
(3) Other causes: vasodilators [Brain's Diseases of the Nervous System. 8th ed. JN Walton. Oxford: Oxford (1977). p 160] and sunbathing [Handbook of Clinical Neurology. **47**: 151 only (1985).].
(4) Re: exercise & vision, see also card EY-603 & [Acta Med Scand. **194**: 161-178 (1954). Takayasu.].
(5) JAMA. **246**: 1113-1114 (1981). Hot bath test caused new signs in 60% of MS patients.
(6) JAMA. **247**: 979 only (1982). Three patients in whom signs did not resolve.
(7) Arch Neurol Psychiat (Chic). **79**: 31-39 (1958). Induced hyperthermia in other neuro diseases.
(8) Multiple Sclerosis. WI McDonald & DH Silberberg. London: Butterworths (1986). pp 117-118.

---

* *neurofibromatosis 1 (NF1)*[1]
* *carotid artery–cavernous sinus fistula, ophthalmic artery aneurysm, orbital cirsoid aneurysm, rapidly growing highly vascular orbital neoplasm*[2]

Abnormally developed craniofacial bones commonly occur in NF1's wide spectrum of clinical manifestations (card FA-003). The most consistent of these dysplasias,[3] hypoplasia of the greater wing of the sphenoid bone, results in an orbit with no posterior wall; only the meninges separate the orbit from the temporal lobe of the brain. In this situation, the temporal lobe will usually herniate into the orbit, causing exophthalmos.[1] Transmission of the brain's normal pulsation[4] to the ocular globe makes the exophthalmos pulsatile.[1] When herniation does not occur, pulsatile enophthalmos may be seen. Either way, the orbit has a "bare" appearance on x-ray.[1]

Other types of meningoencephaloceles may also impart cerebral pulsations to the globe.[1] Transmission of arterial pulsations to the globe occurs in the second group of disorders listed above. Bailey notes that in the first three of these conditions the patient notices a buzzing noise in the head and diminished visual acuity in the affected eye.[2]

(1) New Engl J Med. **311**: 520-527 (1984). CPC on unilateral pulsatile exophthalmos.
(2) Hamilton Bailey's Demonstrations of Physical Signs in Clinical Surgery. 17th ed. A Clain (ed). Bristol, UK: Wright (1986). p 81. "Unilateral pulsating proptosis is a rare condition that always arouses much clinical interest."
(3) Neurofibromatosis. VM Riccardi & JE Eichner. Baltimore: Johns Hopkins (1986). p 137.
(4) In fact, the first written description of the human brain (from the Smith papyrus, circa 2400 BC) is "something throbbing and fluttering under thy fingers." [The Healing Hand. G Majno. Cambridge, MA: Harvard (1975). p 105.]

Eye - Appendages EY-201

Peri-orbital purpura appearing
after proctoscopy, coughing, or vomiting

Eye - External EY-401

Golden-brown or greenish-yellow ring around the iris

Eye - External EY-402

Unilateral arcus cornea

* *amyloidosis*[1]

The maneuvers listed on the obverse all raise intrathoracic pressure and, therefore, venous pressure (by preventing inflow of blood into the thorax). Coupled with the characteristic capillary fragility of amyloidosis,[1] it would not seem surprising that facial capillaries rupture under this pressure load, producing purpura. However, both the external[2] and internal[3] jugular veins have valves that prevent retrograde flow. In the internal jugular vein they are present at least unilaterally in 97% of people[3] and remain competent even with transvalvular gradients of 65 mm Hg.[4] Here, however, the valves may be incompetent, due to chronic congestive heart failure[4] or, conceivably, to amyloid infiltration.

Two other clinical syndromes of hypertensive facial capillary rupture are seen: (1) Peri-orbital petechiae seen in people who [deliberately] hang upside down,[5] and (2) the *masque ecchymotique*, first recognized in persons trampled by a Parisian crowd in 1837[6] and now known as "traumatic asphyxiation";[7] extreme thoracic compression (for example, when a car falls on the chest) plus glottic closure produces striking ecchymoses and engorgement of the head and neck.[6,7]

(1) Mayo Clin Proc. **58**: 665-683 (1983). Clinical and laboratory features of amyloidosis.
(2) Gray's Anatomy. 30th American ed. CD Clemente. Philadelphia: Lea & Febiger (1985). p 816.
(3) Am J Cardiovasc Pathol. **1**: 51-54 (1986). Autopsy study of valve presence.
(4) Circulation. **65**: 188-196 (1982). Competence of jugular venous valves.
(5) New Engl J Med. **307**: 1406-1407 (1982). Letter. "Inversion Therapy," is practiced, of course, using "Gravity Inversion Boots."
(6) The CIBA Collection of Medical Illustrations. FH Netter. Volume 7. Summit, NJ (1979). p 242.
(7) J Trauma. **25**: 838-841 (1985). Long term follow-up after traumatic asphyxia; references.
(–) Whales lack venous valves, leading to stupendous blood loss when harpooned, as vividly described in chapter 81 of Moby-Dick.

(Kayser-Fleischer ring)

* *Wilson disease*
* *non-Wilsonian liver disease*

The term Kayser-Fleischer (KF) ring is reserved for pigmented corneal rings that are shown to contain excess copper in the area of Descemet's membrane (assessed noninvasively by x-ray emission spectrophotometry). They are difficult to see without a slit lamp, and were long thought pathognomonic of Wilson disease.[1]

Recently, however, abnormal copper metabolism and pigmented corneal rings similar to KF rings have been noted in other chronic liver disease, most notably primary biliary cirrhosis (PBC), but also in chronic active hepatitis, cryptogenic cirrhosis, intrahepatic cholestasis of childhood, and partial biliary atresia.[1,2] The highest serum copper level ever reported (3350 mcg/dL; normal, 75 to 145) was in a patient with multiple myeloma and a pigmented corneal ring.[1]

Sometimes the composition of these pigmented rings in non-Wilsonian disease is unclear.[1] In one alcoholic man with cirrhosis the intensity of the rings varied directly with his serum bilirubin concentration.[2] A "pseudo-KF ring" was documented in a patient with carotenemia and pre-existing arcus senilis.[2]

(1) Ann Intern Med. **86**: 285-288 (1977). 3 of 81 PBC patients had pigmented corneal rings.
(2) Arch Intern Med. **141**: 246-247 (1981). Fluctuating KF-like ring.
(–) Color Atlas of the Eye and Systemic Disease. EE Kritzinger & BE Wright. Chicago: Year Book (1984). p 9. Illustration.

---

* *contralateral carotid stenosis*[1]
* *history of homolateral ocular inflammation*[2]

(In discussing this subject, anatomic relations are grasped more quickly if we sometimes refer to the <u>non</u>-arcus side rather than the side with the arcus.)

In the single reported case of unilateral non-arcus owing to homolateral carotid stenosis, the authors postulated that reduced arterial flow prevented the deposition of substances that normally form an arcus. To support this, they noted that unilateral absence of hypertensive and diabetic retinopathy has been seen with homolateral occlusive carotid artery disease.[1]

Unilateral arcus has long been known to occur after homolateral ocular or corneal inflammation[3] (especially if hyperlipidemia is present). The increased vascularity associated with inflammation is probably responsible for the phenomenon.[2]

A 60-year-old man with Wilson disease had unilateral absence of a Kayser-Fleischer ring; he had been blinded in that eye by a penetrating injury at age 7. The consequent reduction of intraocular pressure may have interfered with the diffusion of copper from the aqueous humor into Descemet's membrane.[4]

Do not forget the possibility of a prosthetic eye (card EY-404).

(1) JAMA. **226**: 676 only (1973). Patient also had amaurosis fugax in the non-arcus eye.
(2) JAMA. **238**: 303 only (1977). Like reference 1, a letter.
(3) On the Arcus Senilis. E Canton. London: Robert Hardwicke (1863). pp 2-3.
(4) Quart J Med. **55**: 63-73 (1985). Unilateral Kayser-Fleischer ring.

Eye - External EY-403

Brownish raised plaques
on each side of the limbus

Eye - External EY-404

Jaundiced patient with unilateral scleral icterus

Eye - Motor EY-601

Twitching of eyelids as patient assumes upward gaze

(pigmented pingueculae)

* *Gaucher disease* *(glucosylceramide lipoidosis)*

Pingueculae are visible in normal subjects as raised yellow plaques on each horizontal side of the limbus. Their size increases with age, and they are usually larger on the nasal side (but do not confuse them with Bitot spots). "Brownish pigmentation of the pingueculae occurs as one of the few physical signs in Gaucher disease; the other signs are hepatosplenomegaly and pigmentation of the skin."[1]

Gaucher disease is a relatively common disorder of glycolipid metabolism;[2] excessive accumulation of glycolipid occurs primarily in the reticuloendothelial system. It has been divided into three clinical types:

- **I** chronic non-neuronopathic (or adult) form (McKusick 23080);
- **II** acute neuronopathic (or infantile) form (McKusick 23090);
- **III** subacute neuronopathic (or juvenile) form (McKusick 23100).

Type I may become manifest at any time from birth to old age; bone pain, due to osteoporotic erosion, is a common presenting complaint. It is the type in which pigmented pingueculae have been reported.[3] All three forms are autosomal recessive.

(1) DeGowin & DeGowin's Bedside Diagnostic Examination. 5th ed. RL DeGowin. New York: Macmillan (1987). pp 100, 102.
(2) An estimated 20,000 persons in the United States have it (McKusick 23080.)
(3) The Metabolic Basis of Inherited Disease. 5th ed. JB Stanbury et al (eds). New York: McGraw-Hill (1983). pp 842-856. Comprehensive review of Gaucher disease.

---

* *prosthetic eye*[1]

The incredibly life-like appearance of prosthetic eyes should not be underestimated.[1]

A syndromic association between jaundice and prosthetic eyes also exists: Bailey says "gross enlargement of the liver and a glass eye (which has been worn for, maybe, many years) is practically pathognomonic of secondary melanoma, the primary growth having been in the uveal tract."[2]

Stroke victims may have unilateral jaundice.[3]

(1) DeGowin & DeGowin's Bedside Diagnostic Examination. 5th ed. RL DeGowin. New York: Macmillan (1987). p 85. Amusing story of how life-like prosthetic eyes are.
(2) Hamilton Bailey's Demonstrations of Physical Signs in Clinical Surgery. 17th ed. A Clain (ed). Bristol, UK: Wright (1986). p 239.
(3) Vepfer cited by Fournier (1813) cited by Garrod in Lancet. **I**: 1055 (1928). Can anyone provide more recent references?

(Cogan sign[1])
(twitch response)

* *myasthenia gravis*

The typical twitch response is observable in a myasthenic patient with ptosis. It is usually best demonstrated as the patient slowly moves his or her gaze from downward to upward: As the patient looks upward, the ptotic lid begins to elevate, but can do so for only a fraction of a second before fatiguing and becoming ptotic again. Thus, this transient elevation gives the impression of a twitch.[1,2]

The rapid recovery of myasthenic muscle is similarly illustrated when, after a complete ptosis has been induced by prolonged upward gaze, the patient blinks. The brief relaxation thus afforded the levator palpebrae muscle allows the recovery of at least some of the muscle's function, permitting a partial opening of the lid. If the muscle then fatigues rapidly, the appearance of a twitch again results.[2]

About half of all patients with myasthenia gravis consult an ophthalmologist first and about half of Cogan's myasthenic patients had the twitch response. Aberrant regeneration of nerve III and, in one case, an unexplained tensilon-resistant ophthalmoplegia are other causes of the sign.[1]

(1) Arch Ophthalmol. **74**: 217-221 (1965). Original report; illustrations.
(2) Walsh and Hoyt's Clinical Neuro-Ophthalmology. 4th ed. NR Miller. Baltimore: Williams & Wilkins (1985). pp 844-845. Illustrated.

Eye - Motor EY-602

Infrequent blinking

Eye - Motor EY-603

Patient with rapid, rhythmic nystagmus at all times
who complains of apparent motion of objects

Eye - Motor EY-604

In a dark room or with the eyes closed,
brief flashes of light are seen when the eyes are moved

* *parkinsonism*[1]
* *thyrotoxicosis (Stellwag sign)*[2]

Adults normally blink about 20 times per minute; reading decreases the average to 14. Blinking may occur spontaneously or as part of a reflex (for example, the glabellar tap). Control of the spontaneous rate does not seem solely dependent on ophthalmic factors: blinking 2 to 4 times per minute would maintain the corneal tear film (assuming normal tear production). Light, heat, humidity, corneal anesthesia, blindness, and old age do not affect the rate either.[1]

Infrequent blinking in parkinsonism (11/min) and excessive blinking in schizophrenia (30/min) suggest dopaminergic pathways help govern the blink rate. In both disorders, treatment (with L-dopa and neuroleptics, respectively) moves the rate toward normal. Tardive dyskinesia is also associated with hyper-blinking (32/min),[1] as is the Tourette syndrome.[3] The administration of apomorphine or bromocriptine to monkeys increases their blinking. The author of reference 1 concludes that the blink rate is a useful clinical sign of central dopamine activity.[1]

Memory tasks, strong emotions, forehead tension, and speech also increase blinking. Atropine increases it and physostigmine decreases it, implying there may be a component of cholinergic control as well.[1]

(1) Brain. **106**: 643-653 (1983). Blinking & the dopaminergic system; no mention of thyroid disease.
(2) DeGowin & DeGowin's Bedside Diagnostic Examination. 5th ed. RL DeGowin. New York: Macmillan (1987). p 81.
(3) Hippocrates. **1(4)**: 66-71 (1987). Lay description of Tourette syndrome in a physician.

---

* *occupational nystagmus*[1]

Better known as miners' nystagmus, this now-rare condition afflicted people working in poor illumination, such as miners working on badly lit coal faces. "In dark adaptation the peripheral portions of the retinæ are more sensitive than the macular regions and are therefore employed in preference to central fixation. In order to avoid fatigue no one extramacular point is made use of, but the images of the object at which the miner gazes are switched from point to point on the retinæ by movement of the eyes. These movements eventually become established, even in good illumination."[2]

At first the patient is unaware of the eye movements and has no symptoms. Later, sight loss ensues, most marked at night and when attempting to perform skilled tasks. Subsequently, exertion or stooping causes giddiness and temporary sight loss. Ultimately the patient notices apparent motion of lights and surrounding objects (oscillopsia). Headache, photophobia, head tremor, and a peculiar mental state also occur.[3]

At least 10 years underground are usually required before the disorder develops, and an average of 15 months separates the first symptom and the inability to work. Most patients eventually recover.[3] Lighting in mines is better now.

(1) By contrast, opsoclonus is a rapid, irregular, non-rhythmic eye movement in horizontal and vertical directions [Stedman's Medical Dictionary.]. "It is an alarming and unforgettable clinical finding. The eyes undergo spontaneous conjugate jerking in any linear or rotatory direction at lightning speed, up to 10 times per second" [New Engl J Med. **318**: 563-570 (1988). CPC on opsoclonus.]. Consult a neuro-opthalmology textbook for a full discussion of nystagmus cum oscillopsia.
(2) Introduction to Clinical Neurology. G Holmes. Edinburgh: Churchill Livingstone (1968) pp 116-117.
(3) Occupational Eye Diseases and Injuries. J Minton. London: William Heinemann (1949). pp 99-107. He cites: Br J Ophthalmol. **32**: 193-232 (1948). More on exertion & sight loss: card EY-001.

(movement phosphenes)

* *optic neuritis / multiple sclerosis*[1,2]

As every schoolchild knows, pressing or rubbing the optic globe causes the appearance of bright, transient flecks of light called phosphenes.[3] Normal persons may see them also when the eyes are moved to the extremes of horizontal or vertical gaze.[1] Older myopes see "movement phosphenes" if eye motion causes their degenerated, retracted vitreous humor to tug on the retina.[4]

In demyelinating disease, movement phosphenes are most common shortly after recovery from optic neuritis, but may precede the attack or occur independently of other visual symptoms. They persist for about 6 weeks.[2] Their postulated cause, an abnormal sensitivity to traction on the optic nerve,[1,2] is appealing for two reasons: (1) The optic nerve is one of the two most mobile structures in the central nervous system (the other is the cervical spinal cord);[2] additional traction may result from the origins of the superior and medial rectus muscles, which are both intimately fused with the optic nerve's sheath.[1,5] (2) Movement phosphenes may be the visual equivalent of the better known Lhermitte sign, in which the disagreeable "electric" sensations that pass down the back after neck flexion are thought to result from traction on damaged posterior columns in the cervical spinal cord.[1,2]

(1) Neurology. **26**: 1100-1104 (1976). Nine cases of movement phosphenes in multiple sclerosis.
(2) McAlpine's Multiple Sclerosis. WB Matthews et al. Edinburgh: Churchill Livingstone (1985) p 220.
(3) That is, any schoolchild who has read: Scientific American. **244(5)**: 174-184 (1981).
(4) Neurology. **35**: 1078-1081 (1985). The so-called "Lightning streaks of Moore."
(5) The perioptic arachnoid membrane is similarly fused (reference 1), lending credence to a forgotten student's authoritatively made comment that pain on lateral gaze is a meningismus equivalent.

Eye - Ophthalmoscopy

EY-801

Broad lines of pigment radiating from the optic disk
and
branching in the manner of blood vessels

Family History

FA-001

Congenital complete heart block
in an offspring

Family History

FA-002

Several family members with unilateral
lymphadenopathy

(angioid streaks[1,2])

* *pseudoxanthoma elasticum (PXE)*
* *Paget disease of bone, sickle cell disease, pituitary tumors*[2]
* *familial hyperphosphatemia with metastatic calcification*[2]

PXE is a heritable disorder of elastic tissue also characterized by skin disease, gastrointestinal bleeding, and heart disease (due to vascular calcification). Most patients are unaware of their skin disease, but angioid streaks often blur or distort vision.[3] The streaks result from calcification and cracking in the outer elastic portion of Bruch's membrane and are believed to parallel the lines of force exerted on the membrane by intra- and extraocular muscles.[4]

Half to two thirds of all angioid streaks occur in PXE. Eighty-five percent of PXE patients have them, *vs* 8% to 15% in those with severe cases of Paget disease. One percent of young sicklers have the streaks, but this may rise to about 20% by age 40.[1]

Angioid streaks have been reported both in normal individuals and with many pathologic conditions.[1,2] However, these associations are of uncertain significance,[2] as coincidence or unrecognized PXE could be responsible.[1] It has recently been shown, for example, that the traditional method of diagnosing PXE (biopsy of the characteristic yellow papules and plaques on flexural skin areas) misses some patients with the disease.[5]

(1) Survey Ophthalmol. **26**: 235-246 (1982). Review of angioid streaks.
(2) DM (Disease-a-Month). **30(14)**: 1-64 (1978). An internist looks at fundi. See pp 15-17.
(3) Physicians' Guide to Oculosystemic Diseases. WV Delaney. Oradell, NJ: Medical Economics (1982). pp 356-8.
(4) New Engl J Med. **308**: 579-585 (1983). A CPC on PXE.
(5) New Engl J Med. **317**: 347-350 (1987). Diagnosis by biopsy of scars and normal-appearing skin.

---

* *systemic lupus erythematosus in the mother; neonatal lupus in the offspring*

In its fullest clinical expression, neonatal lupus erythematosus (NLE) is characterized by a transient dermatitis, a variety of transient systemic and hematologic abnormalities, and isolated complete heart block.[1] Probably an underdiagnosed disease, about 150 cases had been reported through 1986.[2] Passive transplacental transfer of auto-antibodies (usually the Ro/SSA or La/SSB antibodies[3]) from mother to fetus seems responsible for NLE,[1,2] although the precise pathogenetic mechanism is still unclear.[4]

The heart block is usually complete and irreversible.[2] Some authors insist it occurs in isolation,[2] whereas others state that structural congenital heart disease is present in 25% of heart-blocked NLE infants and, further, that various other conduction defects may occur instead.[1]

Roughly half of these mothers are asymptomatic at the time their affected infant is delivered. Systemic lupus or another connective tissue disease, such as rheumatoid arthritis or Sjögren syndrome, will develop in most of them months to years later (the record is 16 years).[1] There is a suggestion that, given enough time, all such mothers will become symptomatic.[2] Whether symptomatic or asymptomatic at delivery, the disease in these mothers is usually mild.[2]

(1) Medicine. **63**: 362-378 (1984). Clinical and laboratory review of NLE. See McKusick 23470.
(2) Ann Intern Med. **106**: 518-523 (1987). Maternal and fetal outcome in NLE.
(3) New Engl J Med. **316**: 1135-1138 (1987). Describes a novel auto-antibody type in NLE.
(4) New Engl J Med. **315**: 667-672 (1985). The antibodies may react with fetal cardiac tissue.

---

* *cat scratch disease*[1]

Recently identified as a bacterial infection,[2] cat scratch disease has long been known to occur as micro-epidemics in families. In most such families, from two to five cases develop within a few weeks of each other, although 1-year intervals between cases have been observed. Through 1967, all reported family epidemics had occurred in multi-cat households, "almost always" including a kitten.[3]

Despite the lyrical appellation "Cat Scratch Fever," 40% of patients are afebrile. Indeed, over 75% of patients have a mild illness (generalized aching, malaise, and anorexia), which suggests that the disease is not rare, but underdiagnosed.[2,4] Lymphadenopathy, sometimes suppurative, is a *sine qua non*. It is usually solitary or regional, being bilateral and noncontiguous in less than 2% of cases.[2] A skin test is available.[2]

Although other animals may sometimes act as the vector, 99% of patients report feline contact. In 90% an inoculation site can be identified, and most cases occur in the last 6 months of the year. At least 10% of patients are adults.[2]

(1) "Gram-negative bacilli." RH Rubin et al. In: Scientific American Medicine. E Rubenstein & DD Federman (eds). New York: Scientific American (3/87). 7:II:31-32. Has since been updated.
(2) Am J Dis Child. **139**: 1124-1133 (1985). Summary of 1200 cases.
(3) Prog Med Virol. **9**: 256-301 (1967). Pages 264-265 recount micro-epidemics.
(4) J Infect Dis. **155**: 390-402 (1987). A series of severe cases.
(–) Lancet. **I**: 960-963 (1988). Kaposi sarcoma mimicked by cat scratch disease.

Family History FA-003

Family history of drowning

Family History FA-004

"Yeah, Doc, everybody at home has this miserable winter cold"

General GE-000

Great imitators

* *neurofibromatosis 2 (NF2)*[1]

NF is a heritable, common, serious, and profoundly heterogeneous disorder;[2] from five[3] to eight[2] subtypes may exist. NF1, the von Recklinghausen type, is *chiefly* characterized by café-au-lait spots and cutaneous neurofibromas (see cards TH-011 and EY-002). In NF2, where these manifestations are absent or attenuated, over 95% of patients have bilateral acoustic neuromas.[4] Symptoms usually begin in the teens or early twenties.[4]

Because these tumors arise from the vestibular nerve (card EA-009), bilateral tumors may interrupt all inputs from the vestibular system to the brain. Yet, a history of imbalance or unsteadiness may still be difficult to obtain[4] because, under normal conditions, the visual and proprioceptive senses provide sufficient information to the brain to control posture. In the dark, however, "avestibular" persons must rely on proprioception alone, and may then notice unsteadiness. The situation underwater is even worse for these people, as visual and proprioceptive cues may *both* be absent. Completely unable to tell up from down, suspended in a homogeneous medium devoid of breathable air – one can only imagine the panic that ensues.

(1) R Eldridge, MD. Clinical Center Grand Rounds, National Institutes of Health, 18 Nov. 1987.
(2) Neurofibromatosis. VM Riccardi & JE Eichner. Baltimore: Johns Hopkins (1986). pp 169-183.
(3) Ann NY Acad Sci. **486**: 45-56 (1986). Clinical & genetic aspects of NF. NF2 is autosomal dominant (McKusick 10100).
(4) New Engl J Med. **318**: 684-688 (1988). Clinical aspects of NF2. Co-authored by Eldridge.
(–) Surprisingly, proprioception is arguably the most essential of the three posture-controlling senses; see the fascinating essay on pp 42-52 of: The Man Who Mistook his Wife for a Hat and Other Clinical Tales. OW Sacks. New York: Summit Books (1985).

---

* *carbon monoxide poisoning*

Carbon monoxide (CO) is the leading cause of death from poisoning in the United States. Its major source is the incomplete combustion of organic fuels. Thus, malfunctioning or poorly vented furnaces, water heaters, and space heaters are common home sources of the vapor.[1] Use of gas kitchen stoves for supplemental heat, a frequent practice in urban dwellings, produces significant CO as well, and keeping a pot of water on the burner for humidity control increases the level further, by limiting oxygen to the flame and thereby promoting incomplete combustion.[2]

Headache, dizziness, weakness, nausea, "trouble in thinking," and dyspnea are the most common early symptoms. It is easy to see why "flu-like viral illness" is the most common misdiagnosis: (1) These nonspecific symptoms will arise when cold weather arrives (as CO-producing heating devices are turned on), which usually coincides with the "flu season;" and (2) because of shared exposure, family members will simultaneously be ill. Worse yet, increased body temperature is "not uncommon." Diarrhea may also occur; thus food poisoning is another frequent misdiagnosis.[1]

CO poisoning must be considered in anyone presenting with a flu-like illness.[1] Whether to measure or not measure blood carboxyhemoglobin levels in these patients is not always clear cut; however, ophthalmoscopy can help: Flame-shaped retinal hemorrhages are a sensitive (but nonspecific) indicator of subacute exposure.[3]

(1) Can Med Assoc J. **133**: 392-397 (1985). Review of CO poisoning. Cigarettes make CO, too.
(2) Ann Intern Med. **107**: 174-176 (1987). CO poisoning in patients with headache & dizziness.
(3) JAMA. **239**: 1515-1517 (1978). Illustrated.

Hackneyed as it is, the description "great imitator" can be usefully expanded beyond the greatest of masqueraders (syphilis[1,24]) to other multisystem disorders that should be considered, however briefly, for inclusion in virtually every differential diagnosis.[2]

Infections
- subacute bacterial endocarditis[3]
- Whipple disease[4]
- tuberculosis[5]
- disseminated mycoses[6]
- Lyme disease[7]
- brucellosis[8]

Intravascular disease[9]
- subacute bacterial endocarditis[3]
- cardiac myxoma[10]
- vasculitis[11,12]
- mycotic aneurysm[13]
- aortic dissection[14]
- atheroemboli[15]

Masses and miscellany
- renal cell carcinoma[16]
- lymphoma[17]
- leukemia[18]
- amyloidosis[19]
- poisoning[20]
- others[21]

Multisystem disorders are good imitators because, in theory, dysfunction of any single organ system may be the disease's initial presentation. Later, unusual combinations of organ system dysfunctions may further confuse diagnosis. Thus, detailed knowledge of the natural history of these diseases is important.[22,23]

(1) "...the extraordinary facility with which syphilis apes every disease in any field of medicine." [Modern Clinical Syphilology. 3rd ed. JH Stokes et al. Philadelphia: Saunders (1944). p 41.]
(2) Since the concept of imitation is primarily a subjective one, the subjective nature of the statements below should be expected.
(3)-(24) See next three cards.

General GE-000

Great imitators

(Second of four cards)

General GE-000

Great imitators

(Third of four cards)

General GE-000

Great imitators

(Fourth of four cards)

(references continued from previous card)

(3) "the great masquerader" [Endocarditis. MA Sande et al (eds). New York: Churchill-Livingstone (1984). p vii.]. Cases with minimal signs of infection are especially difficult.

(4) "... a multiplicity of presenting manifestations [make] it a 'great mimic.'" [Whipple's Disease. WO Dobbins III. Springfield, IL: Thomas (1987). p vii.]

(5) "The clinical manifestations of tuberculosis are so varied and subtle that this disease should be kept constantly in mind.... Few diseases with the prevalence of tuberculosis simulate so many other conditions." [reference 22, p 638]

(6) Eg, coccidioidomycosis, "a great 'imitator disease,' comparable with tuberculosis or syphilis in the range of its manifestations." [Arch Pathol Lab Med. **110**: 182 only (1986).]

(7) "... protean manifestations and a tendency to mimic other common diseases" [Ann NY Acad Sci. **539**: xiii-xiv (1988).]. As page 58 of the same volume notes: "There are many obvious similarities between Lyme disease and syphilis. The major ones are their spirochetal etiology, the ability of the spirochetes to stay alive in human tissue for years, occurrence of clinical manifestations in stages, early disease in the skin and later disease in the brain, and susceptibility to antibiotic treatment."

(8) "the signs and symptoms simulate those found in many other conditions of ill-health" [The Nature of Brucellosis. WW Spink. Minneapolis: U. of Minnesota Press (1956). p 191.]. The truism that "few diseases are as often misdiagnosed or remain as long undiagnosed as brucellosis" [Scot Med J. **21**: 132-133 (1976).] is epitomized by the case of the brucellosis expert who realized he had contracted the disease only after seven weeks of illness [Rev Infect Dis. **5**: 821-842 (1983).].

(9) Since intravascular disease can compromise the blood flow to any organ, these conditions have a fearsome imitative ability. It is noteworthy that Philip Tumulty, one of the most astute diagnosticians in the 4000 years of human medicine, concentrated his clinical scholarship on four intravascular diseases: PAN, SLE, GCA, and SBE [Johns Hopkins Med J. **137**: 141 only (1975). Illustrated.].

(10-24) See next two cards.

(references continued from previous card)

(10) "... an extraordinary variety of nonspecific clinical signs and symptoms capable of masquerading as many other ... cardiovascular and systemic diseases." That is, myxomas have both systemic and embolic effects. [Heart Disease. 3rd ed. E Braunwald (ed). Philadelphia: Saunders (1988). pp 1470-1473.]

(11) "Within the entire spectrum of vasculitis virtually any size or type of blood vessel in any organ system can be involved." [Ann Intern Med. **89**: 660-676 (1978).]

(12) Of course, lupus is itself known as a great imitator: "it's numerous clinical presentations have mandated the inclusion of lupus erythematosus in virtually every differential diagnosis." [Systemic Lupus Erythematosus. RG Lahita (ed). New York: Wiley (1987). p xvii].

(13) Though in many cases a complication of infective endocarditis, I feel mycotic aneurysm deserves separate mention because (1) it seems, a priori, capable of producing many of the effects of infective endocarditis, and (2) it may lurk almost anywhere in the body.

(14) "[Aortic dissection] must be considered in every acute condition, not only of the chest, but also in the head, abdomen, and extremities." [Medicine. **37**: 217-279 (1958). 505 dissections.] "Acute condition" can even include sepsis [Arch Surg. **91**: 263-275 (1965). Aneurysm rupture.].

(15) "Multiple atheroemboli can produce any of the features of vasculitis." [New Engl J Med. **315**: 308-315 (1986). A CPC.] Therefore, an imitator of an imitator.

(16) "Renal cell carcinoma has been called the 'internist's tumor.'" [Medicine. **55**: 291-311 (1976).]

(17) Lymphomas may arise in (1) lymphoid tissue, or (2) sites that normally contain no lymphoid tissue (eg, stomach). Thus, they may occur anywhere in the body [Cancer. **29**: 252-260 (1972). Extranodal lymphomas.]. This, then, is also an instance of the fact that neoplasia is "properly considered in virtually every differential diagnosis" [The Principles and Practice of Medicine. 22nd ed. AM Harvey et al (eds). East Norwalk, CT: Appleton & Lange (1988). p 368.].

(18-24) See next card.

(references continued from previous card)

(18) "There is no organ or tissue in the body which has not been involved by leukaemic infiltration, with or without the production of clinical signs and symptoms." [Quart J Med. **9**: 67-91 (1940).]

(19) "There is scarcely a disease in the entire category of our clinical heritage which may not be mimicked by amyloidosis." [Rare Diseases and Lesions. WB Bean. Springfield, IL: Thomas (1967). p 37.]

(20) Example: Carbon monoxide poisoning, which "may rank with syphilis, tuberculosis, and subdural hematoma in its ability to simulate a variety of systemic diseases" [JAMA. **246**: 1698-1700 (1981).]. The gamut of signs and symptoms in heavy metal poisoning are even more daunting; a single article on plumbism is all that's needed to convince: Medicine. **62**: 221-247 (1983).

(21) Sarcoidosis is a "disease of infinite variation" [ref. 19, p 147]. Perhaps extramedullary hematopoiesis belongs on the list because, like lymphoma, it can generate masses almost anywhere. The clinical manifestations of the Munchausen syndrome are limited only by the mind's inventiveness.

(22) Differential Diagnosis. 3rd ed. AM Harvey et al (eds). Philadelphia: Saunders (1979). Pages 611-718 [sic] cover multisystem disorders.

(23) Some imitators specialize in single organ systems. Thus, "multiple sclerosis has supplanted syphilis as the Hydra of clinical neurologic disease" [Handbook of Clinical Neurology. **47**: 49-78 (1985). (p 49)], and chronic subdural hematoma "has been called the 'neurological imitator'" [Quart J Med. **48**: 43-53 (1979).]. AIDS has been similarly dubbed [J Am Geriatr Soc. **35**: 467-468 (1987).], and do not forget Lyme disease (reference 7).

(24) Because of the human immunodeficiency virus, syphilis seems to be entering a "third generation" of imitation in which serologic tests lose their sensitivity [eg, Ann Intern Med. **107**: 492-495 (1987).] and natural luetic history changes drastically [eg, New Engl J Med. **316**: 1569-1572 (1987).]. (The previous generations of syphilitic mimicry are epitomized by, first, the Oslerian cliché "Know syphilis in all its manifestations and relations, and all other things clinical will be added unto you" [New Engl J Med. **316**: 632 only (1987).], and second, by the book: Spirochetes in Late Seronegative Syphilis, Penicillin Notwithstanding. JL Smith. Springfield, IL: Thomas (1969). 343pp.)

General GE-001

Approach to the varied causes of any particular set of symptoms and signs

(mnemonic)

General GE-002

Sets off an airport metal detector,
even after all metallic personal effects are removed

General GE-003

Pulsatile mass
that is not an aneurysm

* *VINDICATE*[1]

V – Vascular
I – Inflammatory / Infectious
N – Neoplastic
D – Degenerative / Deficiency states
I – Intoxication
C – Congenital
A – Autoimmune / Allergic
T – Trauma
E – Endocrine / metabolic

To the above, I would add another "I" – iatrogenic.[2]

(1) Mnemonics, Rhetorics and Poetics for Medics. RL Bloomfield & ET Chandler. Winston-Salem, NC: Harbinger Press (1982). p 2.
(2) Iatrogenic Diseases. 3rd ed. PF D'Arcy & JP Griffin. New York: Oxford (1986). 1086 pp.

---

* *iron overload*

As treatment for a myelodysplastic syndrome, the patient reported had received approximately 300 units of blood over the previous 4 years.[1]

Similarly, two visitors to the White House who had undergone thallium-201 stress tests within the previous 4 days were detained by the Secret Service after the residual radioactivity in their bodies triggered the security alarm there.[2] Bank vaults may have radiation detectors too.[3]

(1) New Engl J Med. **307**: 1459 only (1982). Letter. Do prosthetic joints trigger airport metal detectors? Does shrapnel?
(2) New Engl J Med. **315**: 836-837 (1986). Letter. Neither triggered airport security devices.
(3) New Engl J Med. **319**: 587 only (1988). Alarm set off by a man one day after Tl-201 stress test.

---

* *neoplasm*

"A very rapidly growing vascular neoplasm, particularly a bone sarcoma, often pulsates very obviously. A swelling which has most of the characteristics of, but is not, an aneurysm, is a sarcoma" (the Morison rule).[1]

By contrast, Bean states that bone metastases from renal cell carcinoma are the most common cause of nonaneurysmal pulsatile swelling, having observed 3 instances in 80 cases of the tumor.[2,3] "Rarely other very vascular tumors such as angiosarcomas [and] metastatic lesions from carcinoma of the thyroid may pulsate, especially when lodged in bone."[2]

A mass may *appear* to pulsate when it transmits the pulsation from a contiguous artery, such as the aorta. (But also see card EY-002.) True "expansile" pulsation is demonstrated by placing the hands on the opposite side of the mass and showing that they alternately approach and recede.[4]

(1) Hamilton Bailey's Demonstrations of Physical Signs in Clinical Surgery. 17th ed. A Clain (ed). Bristol, UK: Wright (1986). p 26. See also card TH-009.
(2) Vascular Spiders and Related Lesions of the Skin. WB Bean. Springfield, IL: Thomas (1958) pp 217-218.
(3) DeGowin & DeGowin's Bedside Diagnostic Examination. 5th ed. RL DeGowin. New York: Macmillan (1987). p 462. Renal cell carcinoma.
(4) Ibid. p 516.

General GE-004

Small handwriting

General GE-005

Situs inversus

General GE-006

Patient smells like putrid fish

* *parkinsonism*[1]
* *macropsia;*[1] *hemiplegia and other corticospinal conditions*[1]

First recognized by Arnold Pick in 1903,[1,2] micrographia was discussed in Kinnier Wilson's 1925 Croonian lectures.[1] He defines it as "an obvious reduction in size of the lettering of the writer in comparison with his [pre-morbid] calligraphy," and further requires that the micrographia be as obvious at the beginning of a sentence as at its close.[1] Thus, neither the natural, but "almost microscopic hand" of Emily Brontë, nor an "increasingly smaller lettering due to fatigue or other inability to preserve the original size" satisfy Wilson's definition.[1,2]

Micrographia may be absent in severe cases of parkinsonism, or be pronounced when other manifestations of the disease are minimal. Hemiplegia or monoplegia, apparently of whatever cause (Wilson gives cerebral syphilis and cerebral arteriosclerosis as examples), may produce the "typical form" of micrographia.[1] Macropsia (the perception of objects as larger than they are) and disorders of the kinesthetic sense are additional causes he cites.[1,3] Although Wilson notes that improvement or disappearance of parkinsonian micrographia under hypnosis has been recorded,[1] simpler methods may also be effective.[4]

(1) "Disorders of motility and of muscle tone." Lancet. **II**: 1-10 (1925). Pages 53-62, 169-178, 215-219, and 268-279 complete the lectures. Lacks citations, but reference 2, below, has them.
(2) Neurology. SAK Wilson & AN Bruce. Baltimore: Williams & Wilkins (1940) p 120.
(3) "Dysmetropsia and its pathogenesis." SAK Wilson. Trans Ophthal Soc UK. **36**: 412-444 (1916). Cited by reference 1. Similarly, micropsia causes megalographia.
(4) Rev Neuro. **37**: 635-638 (1921). Use of paper ruled with widely spaced lines; in French.
(–) New Engl J Med. **309**: 375-376 (1983); **316**: 114 only (1986). Discusses Hitler's [parkinsonian?] signature and attempted forgeries. See card GE-008.

---

* *homozygous twin*

Conjoined twins are *not* identical: they are enantiomorphs (like bookends). One of the twins, therefore, always has situs inversus.[1]

This phenomenon is also seen in some nonconjoined homozygous twins. The most famous example is Tweedledum and Tweedledee in Lewis Carroll's *Through the Looking Glass*.[1,2] The twins on NBC-TV's short-lived show "Double Trouble" are also "mirror twins."[3]

A Polish pathologist named Hellin made the interesting observation that twins occur once in every 89 births, triplets once in every 89^2 births (= 1 in 7921), and quadruplets once in every 89^3 births (= 1 in 704,969).[4]

(1) Animal Asymmetry. AC Neville. London: Edward Arnold (1976) pp 20-21.
(2) The Annotated Alice. L Carroll. Annotated by M Gardner. New York: Bramhall House (1960) pp 231-234.
(3) The Tonight Show. NBC-TV. March 28, 1984.
(4) Stedman's Medical Dictionary. Baltimore: Williams & Wilkins (1976). pp 621 & 763. Entered under "law, Hellin's." The numbers are, of course, meant to be approximations.
(–) Barely relevant to this discussion is the observation that "the hazards of being conceived a twin include an increased risk not only of stillbirth and various neurologic abnormalities, but also of being pursued through life by a growing band of twin researchers" [Lancet. **II**: 244-245 (1980).].

---

* *trimethylaminuria*[1]

The only clinical manifestation of this inborn error of metabolism is a foul body odor similar to that of "rotting fish." The psychosocial problems can be considerable; families may tell of several frustrating years of counseling about better body hygiene, and of numerous referrals to specialists.[2]

The odor is due to trimethylamine (TMA). Intestinal bacteria metabolize ingested choline (itself having a fishy odor) to TMA, which is then absorbed and converted to nonodorous TMA-oxide in normal persons, but not in subjects with trimethylaminuria. Dietary restriction of choline leads to marked odor amelioration.

The diagnosis is made by measuring urinary TMA levels after oral loading with choline. The general unavailability of this assay and the lack of physician awareness may contribute to the disorder's apparent rarity. However, the profound beneficial effect of treatment on the patient makes detection important.

Fishy odors are also found in uremia[3] and in zinc oxide users.[4] The production of a fishy odor when potassium hydroxide is added to a vaginal discharge is known as a "positive whiff test" and implicates *Gardnerella vaginalis* as the cause.[5]

(1) Ann Clin Lab Sci. **13**: 20-24 (1983). Clinical and chemical considerations.
(2) JAMA. **251**: 253-255 (1984). Case report.
(3) New Engl J Med. **297**: 132-135 (1977). High TMA concentrations in uremic breath.
(4) The Whole Emergency Medicine Catalog. MS Jastremski et al. Philadelphia: Saunders (1985). pp 16-17.
(5) Medical Knowledge Self-Assessment Program VII. Philadelphia: American College of Physicians (1985). pp 27, 164.

General GE-007

Drives with both hands on the steering wheel

General GE-008

Heroin that causes a burning sensation at the site of injection

GI GI-001

Silver stools

(Fleming sign)

* *universal sign of the bad driver*

Gentle Reader, do not hate me for this card. Here are my reasons for including it:

(1) It is true. Think of your own driving: you *always* have one hand on the wheel. But when the rain gets blindingly heavy or you realize you're going to take that curve too fast – boom! – both hands go onto the wheel; you have reached the limits of your driving skill. Thus, seeing someone driving down a sunny turnpike straightaway with both hands on the wheel indicates that this simple task is as much as the driver can handle.

(2) To emphasize that observations by nonphysicians can be clinically useful. After all, there are other professions that involve close scrutiny of humans. A journalist's sign is on card SK-302; this, however, is a spy's sign.

(3) To get the proper citation. The sign appears *somewhere* in the corpus of James Bond novels written by former intelligence agent Ian Fleming. Any help?[1]

(4) To emphasize that driving habits are a legitimate concern of physicians. The desirability of reducing the horrible toll of automobile accidents should be self-evident.[2]

(1) Fleming has also written of that "infallible badge of the bad driver, a hat clamped firmly on the exact center of [a man's] head" [Goldfinger. I Fleming. New York: Signet (1959) p 53 (chapter 7).]
(2) JAMA. **259**: 76-80 (1988). How physicians can help prevent automobile injuries.

---

* *"synthetic heroin," containing MPTP*[1]

Several heroin users in the San José, California area developed symptoms and signs of acute severe parkinsonism in spring/summer 1982. They each told of using a "new synthetic heroin" for 4 days to 2 months. All of them also noted "a burning sensation when the drug was injected intravenously, a symptom they considered unique." Different, too, were the immediate subjective effects, which were "more dream-like or 'spacey'" than the conventional heroin euphoria. Some patients also experienced disorientation, transient shadowy visual illusions, hallucinations, and visual blurring.

The initial motor symptoms included intermittent jerking of the limbs and/or increasing "slowness" that was replaced in a few days by stiffness, dysphasia, dysphagia, and sometimes a tremor. Progression of stiffness and slowing continued over several days to 3 weeks. Some patients had abrupt episodes of "freezing up."

The agent responsible for the parkinsonian state is MPTP, a byproduct in the synthesis of the potent meperidine/demerol analog MPPP. MPTP's value in research is that it produces a pure parkinsonian state, unlike the other neurotoxins (CO, CS_2, manganese, neuroleptics) that produce parkinsonism mixed with other neurologic disorders.

There is a suggestion that Adolf Hitler's parkinsonism was caused by injections of synthetic opiates![3]

(1) Neurology. **35**: 949-956 (1985). Detailed histories of 7 MPTP-induced parkinsonism cases.
(2) JAMA. **256**: 3061-3063 (1986). Review of the "designer drug" industry.
(3) The Impact of Illness on World Leaders. BE Park. Philadelphia: University of Pennsylvania Press (1986). Pp 149-219 discuss Hitler. See pp 187-188.

---

* *carcinoma of the ampulla of Vater*[1,2]

* *tropical sprue*[2]
* *jaundice of pregnancy plus iron therapy*[1]
* *children convalescing from diarrhea after sulfonamide administration*[2]

Pale, or "acholic," stools are caused by biliary obstruction. When blood is added to an acholic stool, the stool takes on a silver color. Cancers of the ampulla of Vater are classically associated with silver stools because they (1) bleed by virtue of their neoplastic nature, and, (2) obstruct the flow of bile into the intestine by virtue of their anatomic location.

Bailey (in the 13th edition) describes the color as that of "aluminium paint" and says that in jaundiced patients of mature age "it is fairly characteristic of carcinoma of the ampulla of Vater."[2]

(1) JAMA. **242**: 2433 only (1979). Nice color illustration.
(2) Demonstrations of Physical Signs in Clinical Surgery. 13th ed. H Bailey. Baltimore: Williams & Wilkins (1960). p 42.
(–) Color Atlas of Liver Disease. S Sherlock & JA Summerfield. Chicago: Year Book (1979). p 19. Illustration.

GI GI-002

Vomitus types

GI GI-003

Pruritus ani

GI GI-004

Patient claims he can play songs by passing flatus

There are eight kinds of vomitus, according to Bailey:[1a]

1) ingested material as yet unaltered by digestion
2) blood (may be red, partly clotted, or old [coffee ground])
3) gastric juice (clear watery fluid; seen when the patient has not eaten recently)
4) bile (yellow)
5) upper small bowel contents (green)
6) lower small bowel contents ("feculent" – brown and odiferous)
7) feces (rare – signifies gastro-colonic communication or coprophagia)
8) "a peculiar vomit associated with acute dilatation of the stomach," namely a brown-black fluid with myriads of suspended small black particles.[1b] (The vomitus may also be coffee-ground appearing.[2])

(1) Hamilton Bailey's Demonstrations of Physical Signs in Clinical Surgery. 17th ed. A Clain (ed). Bristol, UK: Wright (1986). [a] pp 19-20; [b] p 312. Blue vomitus is discussed on card GI-007.
(2) The Acute Abdomen in Rhyme. 5th ed. Z Cope. London: HK Lewis (1972) pp 95-99. This is an immensely clever book, viz:

And now I'll outline, if I may,
The perforated ulcer play
Which has acts one, two, three, no more
Unless the p.m. be Act 4....
Act One. The patient is at home,
Perhaps doth round the garden roam,
He seems well but for stomach-ache,
Which he puts down to that rich cake
– For that he thinks, without a question,
The cause of all his indigestion –
Then suddenly he gives a cry
And shouts aloud in agony
"My God, I think I'm going to die."
[pp 29-30]

---

* *quinidine, colchicine, mineral oil*
* *ingested irritants: beer, alcohol, coffee, citrus, nuts, popcorn*
* *perianal psoriasis, candidiasis*
* *menopause*

These are true zebras. The overwhelming majority of cases of pruritus ani comes from fecal soiling, fecal leakage, perianal moisture, and local trauma. These conditions have a huge differential. Treatment can be difficult; a set of printed instructions to the patient are considered essential. Pinworms, though an infrequent cause, are reported to have "an awesome if not spectacular" sigmoidoscopic appearance.[1]

By the way, the discovery of pinworm eggs in a 100,000-year-old coprolith makes them the oldest demonstrated infection of humans.[2,3]

(1) Surg Clin North Am. **58**: 505-512 (1978). Practical approach to pruritus ani.
(2) Harrison's Principles of Internal Medicine. 9th ed. KJ Isselbacher et al (eds). New York: McGraw-Hill (1980). p 899. More on pinworms is in: Am Fam Physician. **38(3)**: 159-164 (1988).
(3) Other ancient infections include osteomyelitis in one of the dorsal spines of a 200-million-year-old dimetrodon and dental caries in a 3-million-year-old Australopithecus skeleton. [The Healing Hand. G Majno. Cambridge, MA: Harvard (1975). pp 16-18.
(–) Ann Intern Med. **101**: 837-846 (1984). Pruritus ani and other common anorectal disorders.

---

* *highly developed ability to control anal sphincters*

"An unusual form of 'air sucking' was practiced by the infamous Frenchman, Joseph Pujol (stage name: Le Petomane), who entertained at the Moulin Rouge by 'playing' various tunes via the passage of apparently unlimited quantities of rectal gas. Monsieur Pujol had the unique ability to consciously relax his anal sphincter and simultaneously reduce the intra-abdominal pressure, thus permitting aspiration of gas (or liquid) into the colon."[1]

In their review of flatulence, the authors also note that "Passage of gas per rectum is a much discussed social phenomenon that has received somewhat less scientific study. There appear to be wide individual variations in the composition and volume of gas passed per rectum (from 400 to 2400 mL per day). The number of passages of gas per day in young, normal males averaged about 14 $\pm$ 4 (1 SD)."[1,2,3]

(1) Annu Rev Med. **31**: 127-137 (1980). Review of flatulence.
(2) Gastrointest Endosc. **23**: 41-42 (1976). Explosions during sigmoidoscopy. Cited by reference 1.
(3) Gastroenterology. **12**: 782 (1949). Quantity & quality of flatus. Cited by reference 1.

GI GI-005

In a patient with diarrhea and fecal leukocytes, stool Gram stain shows curved, gram-negative rods arranged as "seagull wings"

GI GI-006

Difficulty flushing stool

GI GI-007

Acutely ill patient whose vomitus etches glass

* *enteritis caused by* Campylobacter jejuni

Half of cases have this finding, which is over 99% specific. Because *C. jejuni* does not grow well on the culture media used for Salmonella and Shigella, and because ampicillin and trimethoprim-sulfamethoxizole are only variably effective, and because the course of the enteritis is not altered if treatment is begun more than 4 to 6 days after onset of symptoms, early diagnosis can be important. Tetracycline is the drug of choice.

Severe cases may mimic inflammatory bowel disease.

(1) Arch Intern Med. **142**: 1858-1860 (1982). Describes the seagull wing sign.
(2) Medical Knowledge Self-Assessment Program VII. Philadelphia: American College of Physicians (1985). p 24. Re-hash of reference 1.
(3) Ann Intern Med. **100**: 615 only (1984). College students, especially men living in university housing, are prone to Campylobacter enteritis.
(4) Ann Intern Med. **98**: 360-365 (1983). Study of 8097 fecal samples for C. jejuni.

---

* *malabsorption*[1]

"Contrary to the common impression that malabsorption or maldigestion produces gross quantities of greasy, oily, rancid-smelling stools, changes in the stool are more often subtle. The most important single feature is the marked difficulty the patient finds in flushing stool because of increased volume and fat content. When fecal fat excretion approaches 20 g/d (normal, less than 6 g/d), at least two flushings are usually required to clear the toilet water."[1]

Another time-honored sign of steatorrhea is the floating stool. Its specificity must be questioned, however, as it is fecal gas, not fat, that causes stools to float.[2]

(1) "Diseases producing malabsorption and maldigestion." GM Gray. In: Scientific American Medicine. E Rubenstein & DD Federman (eds). New York: Scientific American (12/88). 4:XI:1.
(2) New Engl J Med. **286**: 973-975 (1972). Testing why stools float.

---

* *fluoride toxicity*[1]

Ingesting 2 grams of sodium fluoride, an active ingredient of insect poisons, is lethal. Effects of acute ingestion may include:

- tetany – hydrofluoric acid, which is formed when fluoride reacts with gastric acid, combines with calcium to result in hypocalcemia;
- hyperglycemia – due to inhibition of carbohydrate metabolism by fluoride;
- prolongation of the blood clotting time.

It is hydrofluoric acid that etches the glass.[1,2] Chronic ingestion of smaller doses will mottle dental enamel and produce osteosclerosis.[1]

Equally striking inorganic chemical phenomena of the gastrointestinal tract are seen in cases of acute yellow phosphorus poisoning: Smoking and luminescence of vomitus and feces may occur. Classically, these substances will smell like garlic.[3]

(1) DeGowin & DeGowin's Bedside Diagnostic Examination. 5th ed. RL DeGowin. New York: Macmillan (1987). p 910.
(2) Similarly, the touch of someone with cystic fibrosis, whose sweat is chloride-enriched, can be enough to discolor certain silver compounds [New Engl J Med. **255**: 999-1001 (1956).].
(3) JAMA. **235**: 1343-1344 (1976). "Smoking stool syndrome." Some rodenticides contain phosphorus.
(–) Although neither an answer to Carlin's famous question "Where's the blue food?" nor a strictly inorganic reaction, blue vomitus is formed after iodine reacts with starch in the stomach [Clinical Diagnostic Pearls. JC Birnholz & PE Michelson. Flushing, NY: Medical Examination (1971). p 115.].

GI GI-008

Car-sickness as a child

GU GU-001

Painless, macroscopic hematuria
during a minor flu-like illness
or after vigorous exercise

GU GU-002

Pulsatile cervix

* *associated with migraine as an adult*

Motion sickness (which, of course, includes car-sickness) ultimately owes its wretched existence to the vestibular system. Vestibular impairment is frequent in migraineurs:

- 80% have demonstrable vestibular function abnormalities when headache-free;[1]
- about 50% have vestibular symptoms, such as vertigo or giddiness, which may occur either as an aura, with the headache, or during headache-free periods;[2]
- up to 60% had motion sickness in childhood[3] (but cf. reference 4), which may or may not have a forme fruste: childhood "vomiting attacks."[5] Motion sickness in adulthood is also more common in migraineurs than non-migraineurs.[2,4]

Thus, "exaggerated responses to [*passive*] vestibular stimulation is perhaps the commonest, and certainly one of the most incapacitating idiosyncrasies of many migraine patients, and as such they may be shut off from many of the simpler pleasures in life: swings in childhood, roller-coasters in adolescence, and travelling [as a passenger] by bus, train, ship, or plane at all times."[6]

A vasomotor explanation, invoking labyrinthine ischemia, seems the most likely explanation for the motion sickness-migraine association,[1,2] but a metabolic derangement of serotonin metabolism has also been suggested.[2]

(1) Headache. **21**: 110-112 (1981). Study of 1 classical and 19 common migraine patients.
(2) Brain. **107**: 1123-1142 (1984). Study of 200 unselected migraineurs.
(3) Background to Migraine. JN Cumings (ed). New York: Springer (1971). pp 1-7. Study of 450 apparently unselected migraineurs. Chapter is by J Pearce.
(4) Headache. **21**: 227-231 (1981). Normal incidence of childhood car-sickness in 83 migraineurs.
(5) Arch Neurol. **15**: 356-361 (1966). High incidence of childhood vomiting attacks in migraneurs.
(6) Migraine. OW Sacks. Berkeley: University of California Press (1970). pp 162-163.

(synpharyngitic macroscopic hematuria)

* *IgA nephropathy (Berger disease)*

IgA nephropathy is not a rare condition. In most of the world, from 17% to 43% of patients undergoing renal biopsy for primary renal disease have it, although the figure is about 5% in the United States and Britain.[1] It also has been associated with over 20 other diseases.[2] Immunofluorescent staining of glomeruli discloses the characteristic presence of IgA; however, IgA immune complexes are thought to play the pivotal role.[1,2]

Hematuria, often macroscopic and recurrent, is the stereotypical presenting feature. The link with upper respiratory and other mucosal infections (for example, of the gastrointestinal and urinary tracts) apparently stems from the shower of IgA immune complexes generated in response to these infections. (The pathology of some of the 20+ associated diseases, such as celiac disease, includes mucosal defects as well.)[1]

The most frequent presentation is in 10- to 30-year-old males. Once thought a benign condition, as many as 20% of patients will need chronic dialysis or renal transplantation.[1]

Exercise can accentuate hematuria due to glomerular disease;[3] infrequently, it causes gross hematuria in normal persons.[4]

(1) Annu Rev Med. **38**: 157-168 (1987). Recent review. Familial form is McKusick 16195.
(2) Lancet. **I**: 11-14 (1988). Found cytomegaloviral antigen in the glomeruli of 100% of patients.
(3) Campbell's Urology. 5th ed. PC Walsh et al (eds). Philadelphia: Saunders (1986) p 2342.
(4) JAMA. **241**: 391-392 (1979). 1 of 50 marathon runners. March hemoglobinuria is clinically similar [Hematology. 3rd ed. WJ Williams et al (eds). New York: McGraw-Hill (1983) pp 618-619.].
(–) Goodpasture syndrome may present after a viral illness [Diseases of the Kidney. 4th ed. RW Schrier & CW Gottschalk (eds). Boston: Little, Brown (1988) pp 2099-2100.].

(Shelley sign[1])

* *aortic regurgitation*

Many other organs pulsate in aortic regurgitation, yielding more eponymous signs:[1,2]

- Landolfi – pupil
- Müller – uvula
- Gerhardt – spleen
- Rosenbach – liver
- Quincke – subungual capillaries

Thoracic aortic aneurysms may cause similar "pulsating" signs:[3]

- Bozzolo – blood vessels of the nasal mucous membrane
- Drummond – air emerging from the nostrils when the mouth is closed

The Quincke sign is well-known, but is of no diagnostic value, as it is present in most normal individuals (including Quincke himself).[4] Pulsating livers are seen also in right-sided heart disease;[5] recall, too, that expansile pulsation of solid organs must be distinguished from transmitted pulsations (card GE-003).

(1) J Indiana St Med Assoc. **52**: 1283-1289 (1959). Eponyms and physical findings in AR.
(2) Valvular Heart Disease. 2nd ed. JE Dalen & JS Alpert. Boston: Little Brown (1987). p 293.
(3) Stedman's Medical Dictionary. 23rd ed. Baltimore: Williams & Wilkins (1976). See under "sign."
(4) South Med J. **74**: 459-467 (1981). Quincke, de Musset, Duroziez, and Hill signs; see card HD-002.
(5) Essentials of Cardiac Physical Diagnosis. J Abrams. Philadelphia: Lea & Febiger (1987). pp 383-385. Tricuspid regurgitation.

GU GU-003

Scrotal edema
and
left testicular enlargement

GU GU-004

Generalized urticaria, dyspnea, cardiovascular collapse,
and loss of consciousness
in a woman a few minutes after coitus

GU GU-005

Sudden collapse in a pregnant woman,
with the male companion perhaps reluctant to give a history

** left renal vein obstruction*[1] *(for example, by tumor or thrombosis)*

On the right side of the body, the testicular, adrenal, and renal veins normally drain separately and directly into the inferior vena cava (IVC). Not so on the left, where the adrenal and testicular veins empty into the left renal vein, which then empties into the IVC. Thus, proximal obstruction of the left renal vein will also obstruct the left testicular vein, causing the signs noted above. The left renal vein has been called the "vein of the three left paired glands."[2]

Acute onset of a left varicocele has the same pathophysiology and significance, and is classically linked with renal cell carcinoma.[3a,4] Vena caval obstruction or occlusion may produce right-sided or bilateral testiculo-scrotal manifestations.[4]

Asymmetry is present in other male genitourinary disorders, for example, cryptorchidism is more common on the right[5] and idiopathic varicocele on the left.[3a,4,5] Normally the left testis hangs slightly lower than the right; reversal of this situation is said to be a useful clue to the presence of visceral transposition.[3b]

(1) Clinical Diagnostic Pearls. JC Birnholz & PE Michelson. Flushing, NY: Medical Examination (1971). p 35.
(2) Grant's Atlas of Anatomy. 7th ed. JE Anderson. Baltimore: Williams & Wilkins (1978). fig 2-99. The left inferior vena cava disappears during embryogenesis.
(3) Hamilton Bailey's Demonstrations of Physical Signs in Clinical Surgery. 17th ed. A Clain (ed). Bristol, UK: Wright (1986). [a] p 378; [b] p 369 – Ascribes the sign to C. Allan Birch (1903-1983), but I've heard that Osler once used it to make the diagnosis from across the room. True?
(4) Principles of Surgery. 5th ed. SI Schwartz (ed). New York: McGraw-Hill (1989). pp 1734-1735.
(5) Current Surgical Diagnosis & Treatment. 5th ed. JE Dunphy & LW Way. Los Altos, CA: Lange (1981). pp 836, 1036.

** anaphylaxis to seminal fluid*[1]

The symptoms are mediated by IgE antibody; thus a woman may truly be allergic to a man. Hypersensitivity reactions occur over a wide clinical spectrum: In some only a local vulvovaginitis occurs.[2] In several cases (including the anaphylactic one quoted[1]) the hypersensitivity occurred with the woman's first coital experience, suggesting cross-reacting antigen(s). Indeed, many of these patients are atopic.[3]

It is somewhat surprising that such reactions are not more frequent, because, when "viewed from the dispassionate vantage point of immunogenetics[,] coitus in outbred populations entails inoculation of the female ... with a 'cellular' allograft consisting of vast numbers of short-lived haploid cells."[4]

A similar mechanism of disease is illustrated by the penicillin-sensitive woman who had postcoital urticaria only during the time her boyfriend was taking dicloxacillin.[5] (Card TH-202 discusses other cases of venereal drug transfer.) Anaphylaxis to latex condoms can occur.[6]

(1) Immunology. **12**: 247-258 (1967). Report of a dramatic case; she lived. (McKusick 19345)
(2) Clin Allergy. **4**: 249-253 (1974). Spectrum of hypersensitivity reactions.
(3) Ann Intern Med. **94**: 459-465 (1981). Some basic science.
(4) Clinical Aspects of Immunology. 4th ed. PJ Lachmann & DK Peters (eds). Oxford: Blackwell (1982). pp 243, 1110.
(5) JAMA. **254**: 531 only (1985). Postcoital urticaria in a penicillin-sensitive patient.
(6) Internal Medicine News. **21(14)**: 9 only (1988). Quotes JS Taylor at the Noah Worcester Dermatologic Society meeting in Monaco.
(–) Obstet Gynecol. **42**: 138-140 (1973). Xenogeneic anaphylaxis.

** air embolism resulting from orogenital sex*

Even in nonpregnant women, orogenital sex is an established cause of nonsurgical pneumoperitoneum. *Air embolism*, however, has been reported only in pregnant women.[1] In pregnancy, the vagina is extraordinarily distensible: Up to 2 liters of air under pressure may be introduced, which may then dissect through the cervical canal, into the uterus, separate the amniotic membrane from the uterine wall, and gain access to the venous circulation via the subplacental sinuses.[1] Once in the right atrium, air can proceed to the right ventricle (where frothing effectively blocks outflow of blood to the lungs)[2] or squirt through a patent foramen ovale into the arterial circulation (which may lead to a cerebral air embolism).[1] Case histories are dramatic and almost always fatal; perhaps 1% of all maternal deaths are from air embolism.[2]

"The diagnosis is made by auscultation of the heart. A classic 'water wheel' sound is heard."[2] Immediate treatment is to (1) place the patient in a head-down left lateral decubitus position, (2) administer 100% O_2 by the best fitting mask, (3) give high-dose steroids (to decrease cerebral edema) and aspirin (to reduce platelet aggregation), (4) transport to a hyperbaric chamber.[1] Percutaneous aspiration of the right ventricle has also been recommended.[2] The best treatment, however, is prevention. Prenatal care should include specific warning against this practice.[1,2]

(1) Obstet Gynecol. **61**: 653-657 (1983). Review of the 10 cases in the literature; first survivor.
(2) J Indiana St Med Assoc. **74**: 30-32 (1981). Four cases of antepartum air embolism.

GU GU-006

Tissue from transurethral prostatectomy shows endometrial carcinoma

---

GU GU-007

Eosinophils in the urine

GU GU-008

Man with bizarre behavior, complaining of pain in the penis

* *endometrial carcinoma of the prostate*

Because the histology of these tumors is "strikingly" similar to that of endometrial carcinoma of the uterus, they were thought to arise from the utricle, a small diverticulum in the wall of the prostatic urethra that is a remnant of the caudal part of the Müllerian ducts.[2,3] (Recall that in female embryos, the Müllerian ducts develop into the uterus and other sex-related structures, whereas in male embryos, they degenerate almost completely.[4])

The utricle's central location explains why bladder outlet obstruction and hematuria are early symptoms of the tumor, and also why rectal examination and needle biopsy are usually unrevealing. However, it also ensures complete destruction of the utricle during transurethral prostatectomy and makes utricular origin of the tumor difficult to prove.[2,3] Thus, the tumor is currently felt to arise from prostatic ducts and is now called "endometrioid carcinoma of the prostate."[1] Interestingly, it appears responsive to the usual hormonal manipulations aimed at standard "male" prostatic tumors.[1]

In women, remnants of the "male" Wolffian duct may produce a Gärtner cyst in the vaginal or uterine wall.[4] Leydig-Sertoli cell tumors can also occur in women.[2]

(1) Campbell's Urology. 5th ed. PC Walsh et al (eds). Philadelphia: Saunders (1986). p 1473.
(2) Uncommon Malignant Tumors. J Antionades. New York: Masson (1980). pp 180-181, 365-368.
(3) Cancer. **37**: 2255-2262 (1976). Discussion of pathology.
(4) Medical Embryology. 3rd ed. J Langman. Baltimore: Williams & Wilkins (1975). pp 180-185.

(eosinophiluria)

* *acute interstitial nephritis*
* *rapidly progressive glomerulonephritis (RPGN)*
* *acute prostatitis*

Anyone who has tried using Wright stain to detect eosinophils in urine will attest to the difficulty and poor performance of the technique.[1] Recently, however, Hansel stain (originally developed to identify eosinophils in bodily secretions) was shown to substantially improve the recognition of eosinophiluria.[2]

As a result, the clinical spectrum of diseases that cause eosinophiluria is becoming better defined. In 92 roughly consecutive patients with active urinary sediments seen by renal consultants over 1 year, the prevalence of eosinophiluria in various conditions was: interstitial nephritis (10 of 11 patients), RPGN (4 of 10), acute prostatitis (6 of 10), postinfectious glomerulonephritis (1 of 6), acute cystitis (1 of 15), acute pyelonephritis (0 of 10), and acute tubular necrosis (0 of 30).[2]

By contrast, Wright stain showed eosinophils in only 2 of the 11 patients with interstitial nephritis. Three eosinophiluric patients with RPGN who had renal biopsies all had severe interstitial inflammation accompanying the glomerular lesion. Note that eosinophiluria was highly discriminant between interstitial nephritis and acute tubular necrosis in this study population.[2]

(1) J Sotos, personal experience (~10 attempts). [Adding human plasma to the slide doesn't help.]
(2) New Engl J Med. **315**: 1516-1519 (1986). The staining technique takes about two minutes.
(–) New Engl J Med. **315**: 308-315 (1986). CPC; atheroembolism also causes eosinophiluria.

---

* *rabies*[1,2,3]

At least three such cases have been reported. A 22-year-old man complained of generalized body pain, worst in the lumbosacrum and right leg, 3 months after being bitten on the right leg by a dog in Pakistan. He seemed hysterical: "He was exceedingly restless, sweating profusely and rolling about intermittently in agony. At times he sat up in bed holding his penis."[1] Rabies was confirmed at postmortem.

In the other two cases the diagnosis was made clinically. One of these victims also complained of leg pain; neither case mentioned a history of animal bite.

After a variable incubation period (7 days to 19 years (!), but usually 18 to 60 days), the prodromal phase of rabies begins with pain and paresthesias at the site of the bite. If the bite was on a limb, these symptoms may spread proximally (as in case 1, above). Irritability, apprehension, GI and respiratory symptoms, and a sense of impending doom follow. Finally, the acute neurologic phase comes, with its marked hyperactivity, hyperventilation, confusion, and other CNS signs.[4] A paralytic presentation, called "dumb rabies" also exists.[5] No matter the presentation, death is inevitable. (See card HD-305)

(1) Br Med J. **2**: 167-168 (1964). Case report.
(2) Br Med J. **2**: 880 only (1965). Letter from Nigeria; also reports a "tentative" additional case.
(3) Br Med J. **1**: 108 only (1966). Letter from Sri Lanka. Dysuria, leg pain, and wrist pain were also present, initially suggesting a diagnosis of Reiter syndrome.
(4) Principles and Practice of Infectious Disease. 2nd ed. GL Mandell et al (eds). New York: Wiley (1985) pp 898-909.
(5) Trans Roy Soc Trop Med Hyg. **70**: 188-195 (1976). Clinical picture of rabies in man.
(–) Br J Urol. **58**: 224 only (1986). Penile hyperexcitability after a thigh bite.

GU GU-009

Horn projecting from the tip of the glans penis

GU GU-010

Urine stain that darkens after washing

GU GU-011

Palpitation and piercing headache
just before, during, or after micturition

* *cutaneous horn of the penis*[1,2]

In the case reported (the 18th in the English literature), a 1.7 by 0.8 cm^2 hard, cornified cutaneous horn was removed from the glans penis of an 84-year-old man who had undergone circumcision 5 years earlier to correct phimosis. Histologic examination disclosed squamous cell carcinoma.[1,2]

Cutaneous horns are projections of keratinized material arising from the skin. Though usually found on the face, ears, and other light-exposed areas of the body, they may occur anywhere on the skin. The lesions are hard and conical in shape, resembling the horn of an animal, with a bulging erythematous base. All such lesions should be biopsied.[2]

On the penis, cutaneous horns usually appear after adult circumcision for long-standing phimosis, and may be unusual presentations for squamous cell carcinoma of the penis. One third of reported penile horns have been malignant.

Not only may humans have horns, but tails as well.[3]

(1) 1986 Year Book of Dermatology. AJ Sober & TB Fitzpatrick. Chicago: Year Book (1986). Illustrated.
(2) J Am Acad Dermatol. **13**: 369-373 (1985). Cited by reference 1.
(3) New Engl J Med. **306**: 1212-1215; **307**: 1089 only (1982). Tales of tails.

---

* *alkaptonuria*

Alkaptonuria is a heritable, autosomal recessive defect in the metabolism of homogentisic acid. A metabolite of phenylalanine and tyrosine, it both accumulates in tissues (causing the syndrome of ochronosis) and is excreted in the urine. If urine containing homogentisic acid is allowed to stand for some time, it will gradually darken downward from the surface as the acid is oxidized into a dark-brown melanin-like polymer. Alkali speeds this polymerization, which explains why washing the diapers of alkaptonuric infants with soap tends to make the stains more intense instead of removing them.[1] In fact, in Slovakia[2] where, like the Dominican Republic,[3] the disease is relatively common, discolored diapers hanging out to dry help guide investigators to the homes of alkaptonuric children. Alkaptonuric urine will not darken for many hours if it remains acidic. Some patients never notice a urinary color abnormality.[1,4] The pigment also appears in cerumen[2] and in sweat, and can stain the axillary and/or genital skin and clothing.[1,2]

The pigment has an affinity for connective tissue, where it takes a gray to bluish-black hue and may be visible in the ear cartilage and the sclerae. Arthritis, especially of the spine, and cardiovascular disease are the important complications of the disease.[1,2,4]

(1) The Metabolic Basis of Inherited Disease. 4th ed. JB Stanbury et al (eds). New York: McGraw-Hill (1978). pp 268-282.
(2) Johns Hopkins Med J. **145**: 217-226 (1979). 1 in 25,000 Slovaks has alkaptonuria.
(3) McKusick 20350.
(4) Ann Intern Med. **104**: 446 only (1986). Newly diagnosed alkaptonuria in a 70 year old woman with aortic stenosis.

---

* *pheochromocytoma of the bladder*

Physical manipulation of a pheochromocytoma, whether in the operating room,[1] at the bedside,[2] in the bathroom (due to bladder distention or contraction), or in the bedroom,[3] can unleash the classical pheochromocytoma triad of headache, sweating, and palpitations.[4]

Although 95% of pheochromocytomas occur in the adrenals, they may arise from anywhere the paraganglionic system extends, namely from the carotid body to the pelvic floor.[5] By 1980 about 100 cases of bladder pheochromocytomas had been reported.[6] Despite the striking symptoms produced by bladder distention or contraction (which may also include syncope,[7] angina,[6] and profuse sweating), at presentation 50% of patients have normal levels of urinary catecholamines and one third are normotensive.[7,8] Measuring these variables during and after micturition may be diagnostic.[7]

The tumors are usually located submucosally. When they bulge into the bladder lumen and ulcerate, gross, intermittent, terminal hematuria may appear. About 80% are visible at cystoscopy.[8]

(1) Am J Cardiol. **40**: 820-824 (1977). A very severe case, and review of 35 cases.
(2) Eg, flank palpation & adrenal pheo (ref. 4), or bimanual examination & bladder pheo (ref. 3).
(3) This is rare, but it can occur with intercourse and a bladder pheochromocytoma (reference 1).
(4) Clinical Hypertension. 4th ed. NM Kaplan. Baltimore: Williams & Wilkins (1986). pp 375-397.
(5) Am J Med. **78**: 307-316 (1985). CPC on bladder pheochromocytoma.
(6) So Afr Med J. **71**: 178-179 (1987). Case report.
(7) JAMA. **247**: 1863-1864 (1982). Case report.
(8) Pheochromocytoma. WM Manger & RW Gifford Jr. New York: Springer (1977). pp 110-114.

Head HD-001

Rhythmic clicking sounds emanating from the head, unrelated to heart beat

---

Head HD-002

Slight involuntary rhythmic head nodding, synchronous with heart beat

---

Head HD-003

“Fontanelle” in an adult

(eustachian tinnitus[1])

* *palatal myoclonus*

The clicking is the sound of the eustachian tube popping open.[1] Palatal myoclonus is the continuous rhythmic or dysrhythmic movement of the soft palate (40 to 250 times/min), sometimes accompanied by synchronous movements of other structures such as the face, pharynx, larynx, diaphragm, or even extremities.

It is generally believed to be a late complication of a lesion in the dentato-olivary tract, typically developing 6 to 8 months after the acute event, and persisting for life.[2] The main pathologic finding has been hypertrophic degeneration of the inferior olivary nucleus. Thus, palatal myoclonus should not be considered a disease, but a sign of brainstem dysfunction.[3] Underlying causes are diverse: ischemic infarcts, trauma, tumor, multiple sclerosis, aneurysm in the posterior circulation, syphilis, and other degenerative processes.[3]

In more subtle cases of eustachian tinnitus, auscultation over the external ear canal or maxillary sinuses may demonstrate the sound.[4] Patients may complain of "ticking" or "cricket" noises in the ear.[1,5] In some instances the noise and the myoclonus will vanish when the patient opens his or her mouth, making it all too easy to miss the diagnosis. Some patients have voluntary control over the myoclonus.[5]

(1) J Neurol Sci. **5**: 473-492 (1967). Case reports; see especially numbers 9, 13, and 16.
(2) Brain. **109**: 431-441 (1986). Oculopalatal myoclonus.
(3) Arch Neurol. **40**: 155-158 (1983). Palatal myoclonus.
(4) JAMA. **245**: 1146-1147 (1981). Ingenious method to auscultate ear canals.
(5) Acta Oto-Laryn. **Suppl. 116**: 39-45 (1954). More fascinating case reports. See also card HE-301.

(de Musset sign[1])

* *aortic regurgitation*[2]

* *aortic arch aneurysm*[2]
* *massive left pleural effusion*[2]

This sign is named after a patient, the syphilitic French poet Alfred de Musset (1810-1857). It was first noticed by his brother Paul at the lunch table one day in March 1842 and was published in his biography of Alfred.

The sign is of low specificity.[1] Apparently everyone's head bobs somewhat: A physician whose vestibular system was destroyed by streptomycin found that the pulse-beat in his head was sufficient to make the letters on a printed page "jump and blur" as he tried to read.[3]

Head *swaying* (lateral movements) is said to indicate severe tricuspid regurgitation.[4]

(1) South Med J. **74**: 459-467 (1981). Brief review of de Musset sign. See card GU-002.
(2) Presse Med. **8(2)**: 335-337 (1900). Other causes of the sign. In French.
(3) New Engl J Med. **246**: 458-460 (1952). Living without a vestibular system.
(4) Essentials of Cardiac Physical Diagnosis. J Abrams. Philadelphia: Lea & Febiger (1987). p 388.

---

* *treated multiple myeloma*[1]
* *hereditary large parietal foramina*[2]

Plasmacytomas can sometimes be palpated on the skull. During treatment they may become softer, then disappear, leaving only a "pseudofontanelle."[1]

Present in 30% to 45% of the population,[3] the parietal foramina are two small defects in the skull, located just off the midline, that serve as passages for arteries and veins.[4] For reasons unknown, they will sometimes be large enough to be readily palpable (eg, a 1-by-2 cm^2 foramen in a 22-year-old woman[2]). This trait acquired the name "Catlin mark" when it was observed in 16 members of the Catlin family early in this century.[5]

Large parietal foramina are asymptomatic unless forcibly pressed on,[2] but they can be used successfully for malingering.[6,7] It is unclear if the resemblance between Catlin marks and trephinated skulls is sufficient to confuse archeological diagnosis.[2,8]

(1) JAMA. **245**: 2298 only (1981). Letter. Presumably, other causes of lytic skull lesions (such as eosinophilic granuloma, sarcoidosis, osteomyelitis, gummata) could also exhibit this behavior.
(2) Proc Roy Soc Med. **29**: 122-125 (1935). Three hereditary cases, reported by Parkes Weber.
(3) J Anat. **63**: 172-174 (1928-1929). Two cases of large parietal foramina.
(4) Grant's Atlas of Anatomy. 7th ed. JE Anderson. Baltimore: Williams & Wilkins (1978). fig. 7-9.
(5) McKusick 16850, 10760.
(6) Edin Med J. **35(NS)**: 629 (1927). Cited by Weber (reference 2).
(7) And let's not forget "the well-known story of that beggar in the streets of Paris who would allow passers by – for a monetary consideration – to press upon his exposed brain and so causing him to pass out" [The Divine Banquet of the Braine. M Critchley. New York: Raven (1979). p 72.].
(8) Science. **170**: 732-734 (1970). Trephining in North America.
(–) Chronic intracranial hypertension may cause expansion of cranial sutures. [Cerebrospinal Fluid in Diseases of the Nervous System. RA Fishman. Philadelphia: Saunders (1980). p 66.]

Head - Face HD-301

Central portion of frontalis muscle less mobile than more lateral portions

Head - Face HD-302

Painless discharging sinus on the point of the chin, near the midline

Head - Face HD-303

Cheek lesion in the mother of an infant

(Monrad-Krohn sign[1,2])

** Hansen disease*

Certain characteristics of *Mycobacterium leprae* cause the cooler areas of the body to be affected first in Hansen disease. This includes the tips of the ears, some parts of the forehead, the malar regions, the testes, and so forth. In the case of the Monrad-Krohn sign, the small branches of the facial nerve which course medially over the (relatively cool) zygoma to the frontalis muscle are affected, whereas the more lateral portions are spared. The central part of the frontalis is thereby less mobile.[1,2,3,4]

Cards EA-006 and EA-008 describe other thermocranial phenomena. The relatively lower temperature of the pinnae may partially explain the tendency for gouty tophi to form there.[5]

(1) Peripheral Neuropathy. PJ Dyck (ed). Philadelphia: Saunders (1975). pp 1180-1181.
(2) New Engl J Med. **300**: 546-553 (1979). CPC on Hansen disease.
(3) Perhaps also relevant is the fact that "the forehead and scalp are not susceptible to the sort of vasoconstrictor reflexes that are seen in the hands and feet" [Mechanism and Management of Headache. 3rd ed. JW Lance. London-Boston: Butterworths (1978). p 8.].
(4) If, to assess frontalis mobility, you look for forehead wrinkling when the patient gazes upward, beware. Absence of forehead wrinkling with upward gaze is the Joffroy sign of thyrotoxicosis [DeGowin & DeGowin's Bedside Diagnostic Examination. 5th ed. RL DeGowin. New York: Macmillan (1987). p 82].
(5) Arthritis Rheum. **15**: 189-192 (1972). Temperature and the solubility of uric acid.

(median mental sinus)

** root abscess of lower incisors*

Recall that the lower jaw is actually two separate bones joined in the midline. Thus, pus from a root abscess of the lower incisors will track between the two halves of the mandible, then through the skin. X-rays of the mandible are normal and the teeth often appear to be sound when they are examined. Dental x-rays, however, show an area of rarefaction around the roots.[1]

Although Bailey classifies median mental sinus in the small group of disorders amenable to a "snap" diagnosis, clinicians unfamiliar with this condition almost invariably diagnose an infected sebaceous cyst.[1,2]

Root abscess (also known as periapical abscess) may be a cause of fever of unknown origin.[3,4]

(1) Hamilton Bailey's Demonstrations of Physical Signs in Clinical Surgery. 17th ed. A Clain (ed). Bristol, UK: Wright (1986). p 98. Illustrated, including radiograph.
(2) "Pits, fistulas, and sinuses [of the head and neck] may readily be misdiagnosed if the clinician fails to employ a systematic diagnostic approach" [Differential Diagnosis of Oral Lesions. 3rd ed. NK Wood & PW Goaz. St. Louis: Mosby (1985) p 199. Pp 193-203 survey the topic.].
(3) Isr J Med Sci. **21**: 995-998 (1985). Occult facial infections and fever of unknown origin.
(4) Am J Med. **66**: 463-467 (1979). Fever of unknown origin and teeth.

** accidental vaccinia*[1]

Immunization of the infant against the variola virus is done by administering vaccinia virus to the upper arm. At the vaccination site a skin lesion develops within 3 to 4 days that then passes through stages as a papule, vesicle, and pustule (the "jennerian take"), before forming a scab (about day 20) and finally a scar.[2] If the mother (or anyone else) carries the baby so the vaccinated area contacts her cheek during one of the contagious stages, she may be inoculated with vaccinia, then have a jennerian take on her cheek.

Although immunization against the variola virus (smallpox) is today quite rare, the vaccinia virus will probably soon be used as a vehicle to carry a new generation of immunizations.[3]

(1) Hamilton Bailey's Demonstrations of Physical Signs in Clinical Surgery. 16th ed. A Clain (ed). Bristol, UK: Wright (1980). pp 91-92. Illustration.
(2) Medical Microbiology and Infectious Diseases. A Braude. Philadelphia: Saunders (1981). pp 1684-1686.
(3) Annu Rev Immunol. **5**: 305-324 (1987). Vaccinia's role in future immunizations.
(–) Interestingly, it has been recommended that archeologists be vaccinated against smallpox, as viable virus is capable of surviving for many years in the dried scabs of previous victims. Cool, dry conditions (epitomized by burial in permafrost) are especially hospitable for the virus [Lancet. **I**: 1103 only (1985).].

Head - Face HD-304

Mexican woman who claims to have found a way to look younger,
and whose friends agree with her

Head - Face HD-305

Terror and muscle spasms,
provoked by blowing a gentle stream of air onto the face

Head - Face HD-306

Elderly man with
two soft hyperpigmented nodules on the forehead

* *diffuse lepromatous leprosy*[1]

Of the five types of Hansen disease, the one characteristically seen in Mexico (and, to some extent, Central America) is the diffuse lepromatous form. The organisms grow freely in the tissue, particularly just below the skin. "It is called 'pretty leprosy' in Mexico because it tends to iron out the wrinkles in the skin, restoring a youthful appearance to a middle-aged person. Thickening of the skin is apparent if comparative photographs are examined, but no ulcers or granulomas are present."

Among other effects, the vitamin A derivative tretinoin thickens the epidermis and removes fine wrinkles.[2] Reduced skin wrinkling and "a relatively youthful appearance" are said to result from selective dysfunction of the sympathetic nervous system.[3]

(1) New Engl J Med. **300**: 546-553 (1979). CPC on Hansen disease.
(2) JAMA. **259**: 527-532 (1988). Effects of topical tretinoin on photoaged skin.
(3) "Clinical pharmacology: assessment of autonomic function." DB Robertson. Pp 86-101 in: Clinical Diagnostic Manual for the House Officer. KL Baughman & BM Greene (eds). Baltimore: Williams & Wilkins (1981). Card EX-205 links wrinkling and the sympathetic nervous system.

(aerophobia)

* *rabies*

Aerophobia is similar to hydrophobia, but may be "more diagnostic."[1] Hydrophobia does not occur in the paralytic, "dumb" form of rabies, but is present in 17% to 50% of classical, "furious" rabies as part of the disease's acute neurologic phase (card GU-008). Water triggers an overwhelming terror and a violent motor reaction: The inspiratory muscles go into spasm for 5 to 15 seconds, facial muscles contract into a grimace, the neck and back are extended, the arms are thrown up, and there is extreme central nervous system arousal that may lead to convulsions, during which 30% of rabies patients may die. Initially, the hydrophobic response follows attempts to swallow liquid, but later the sight, sound, or even mention of water may trigger it.[2,3]

Rabies encephalitis typically features severe brainstem involvement with relative sparing of the higher cortical centers. It is thought that destruction of the inhibitory centers associated with airway-protecting reflexes (such as the cough, sneeze, aspiration, and immersion reflexes) causes the motor response, and that exaggeration of the normal arousal associated with these basic survival reflexes causes the terror.[2]

Of note, in 20% of the 45 cases of rabies that occurred in the U.S. between 1960 and 1984, no history of animal bite could be elicited.[4]

(1) Per the CDC rabies chief. [Dartmouth Medical School Alumni Magazine, fall 1985, pp 21-23, 35.]
(2) Trans Roy Soc Trop Med Hyg. **70**: 188-195 (1976). Clinical picture of rabies in man.
(3) In fact, the Roman neurologist Cælius Aurelianus cautioned that rabid patients being bled must be prevented from hearing the sound of blood draining into the pan! [The Nature and Treatment of Rabies or Hydrophobia. 2nd ed. TM Dolan. London: Ballière, Tindall, and Cox (1879). p 136.]
(4) Ann Intern Med. **102**: I-123 only (1985). See also Ann Intern Med. **109**: 935-937 (1988).

(prayer nodules[1])

* *Shi'ite Muslim*

Shi'ite Muslims will, in the course of their prayers, rest their head on a flat, baked clay tablet called a "prayer stone." In a single day the forehead will touch the stone more than 30 times, for durations ranging from 5 to 20 seconds. In Iran, where 93% of the population are Shi'ites, the elderly male Muslim "frequently" has two small soft nodules 1 to 1.5 cm in diameter on the forehead, most commonly about 2 cm above the medial ends of the eyebrows. "When these develop he is regarded with additional respect."[1] President Sadat of Egypt had a prayer nodule.[2] Hyperpigmentation and lichenification appear to occur before formation of the nodule.[1]

Sun exposure seems to be an important factor in the development of prayer nodules. Women seldom have prayer nodules, possibly because devout Iranian women who pray frequently do not get exposed to the sun (they either stay predominantly indoors or keep their face covered with a long cloth when they go outdoors).[1,3] A prayer nodule was noted on the left lateral malleolus of a 28-year-old Shi'ite man (Shi'ites sit on their left ankle during part of their prayers).[2,4]

(1) Clin Exp Derm. **4**: 39-47 (1979). Clinico-sociological description.
(2) 1985 Year Book of Dermatology. AJ Sober & TB Fitzpatrick (eds). Chicago: Year Book (1985) pp 322-323. However, I am told Sadat was a Sunni Muslim.
(3) Clin Exp Derm. **7**: 225-226 (1982). Prayer nodule in a woman not habitually covering her face.
(4) Clin Exp Derm. **9**: 97-98 (1984). Yoga enthusiasts may also have nodules on their feet.
(–) The "Mohammedan prayer position" may be spontaneously assumed by patients suffering the pain of chronic pancreatitis [Presse Med. **67**: 1543-1546 (1959). Illustrated.].

Head - Face HD-307

Nontraumatic numbness of the chin

Heart HE-001

Compared to the normal pulse, diminished or unchanged strength of the beat after a premature ventricular contraction

Heart HE-002

Failure of a permanent demand pacemaker during surgery

** cancer*

With the many non-neoplastic cases of facial numbness, it is unusual for symptoms to be restricted solely to the distribution of the mental nerve. Isolated mental neuropathy, the "syndrome of the numb chin," has been associated with a variety of systemic cancers. Although in most reports the diagnosis of cancer precedes the development of numbness, the reference lists nine cases where the opposite occurred. Numb chin may also develop when a treated, known cancer relapses.

Mental nerve palsy is manifested by ipsilateral numbness of the skin of the lower lip and chin and mucous membrane of the inside of the lip, extending to the midline. Jaw metastases with local bone destruction account for most of the cases of numb chin syndrome, but in many cases the cause will be indeterminate after radiographic study. Bone marrow infiltration should also be considered: In nine cancer patients who presented with numb chin (mentioned above), bone marrow biopsy led to the diagnosis in eight.

Neurology. **31**: 1277-1281 (1981). Nineteen cases. Lymphoma (6 patients), leukemia (2 patients), and breast cancer (3 of the 5 women) were the most common tumors found.

(Brockenbrough sign[1])

** idiopathic hypertrophic subaortic stenosis (IHSS)*

The prolonged diastolic period after a premature ventricular contraction ("compensatory pause") normally results in increased filling of the left ventricle and, therefore, a greater left ventricular end-diastolic volume. In accordance with the Frank-Starling mechanism, this causes a greater force of ventricular contraction.[2]

In patients with a fixed resistance to outflow (*eg*, normals, valvular AS, discrete subvalvular AS), the arterial pulse pressure rises as the force of LV contraction rises. In IHSS, however, the size of the outflow orifice is reduced during systole by contracting, hypertrophic myocardium.[3] "If the severity of obstruction were a function of the strength of contraction," as Brockenbrough *et al* surmise, increasing contractile force would increase the stenosis and thus diminish the stroke volume and pulse pressure.[1,4] Alternatively, a long diastole could cause a lower *aortic* end-diastolic pressure, resulting in a less distended, hence higher resistance, LV outflow tract for the next systolic contraction.[5]

This sign (which occurs in one third of IHSS patients)[5] has not been reported as detectable by palpation; it was originally observed with arterial pressure tracings. However, an auscultatory analog seems to exist.[6]

(1) Circulation. **23**: 189-194 (1961). Original report.
(2) Alterations in cardiac calcium kinetics play an additional, if not dominant, role [Heart Disease. 3rd ed. E Braunwald (ed). Philadelphia: Saunders (1988). pp 412-413.].
(3) This is a gross simplification not accepted by all. See: Circulation. **75**: 311-322 (1987).
(4) The pulse pressure may also just stay the same.
(5) Bedside Cardiology. 3rd ed. J Constant. Boston: Little, Brown (1985). pp 43-44.
(6) Ann Intern Med. **104**: 772-776 (1986). Post-extrasystolic murmurs tend not to intensify in IHSS.

** electromagnetic interference from electrocautery*

Electromagnetic interference can confuse the sensing circuits of demand pacemakers, resulting in failure to pace.[1] "The likelihood of this can be reduced by placing the indifferent plate of the cautery unit as far as possible from the head and pulse generator of the permanent pacemaker. In addition, electrocautery should be used in brief bursts rather than continuously. Finally, a magnet should be available in the operating room to convert the pacemaker from the demand to the fixed-rate mode should that be necessary."[2,3]

Cochlear implants are also susceptible to electromagnetic interference.[4]

(1) Anesthesiology. **46**: 127-131 (1977). Perioperative management of pacemaker patients.
(2) Medical Knowledge Self-Assessment Program VII. Philadelphia: American College of Physicians (1985). p 438.
(3) Similarly, implantable defibrillators are routinely turned off just before surgery.
(4) New Engl J Med. **313**: 387 only (1985). Letter; card EA-004 lists other electromagnetic syndromes.
(–) A somewhat more bizarre health complication of a pacemaker occurred in Anglican Church envoy Terry Waite while a hostage in Lebanon. He sustained "serious injuries" when his captors "mistook his pacemaker for a secret transmitter." [Stanford Daily. **193(15)**: 3 (22 Feb 1988).]

Heart HE-003

Suspected tumor in a patient with congenital cyanosis

Heart HE-004

Palpitation followed by polyuria

Heart HE-005

Pulmonary edema
and
perspiration over the forehead, chest, and abdomen

* *pheochromocytoma*[1,2]
* *carotid body tumor (chemodectoma)*[3]

Living at high altitude is known to predispose to the development of carotid body tumors. A similar hypoxemic state may be duplicated at sea level by cyanotic states. Like chemodectomas, pheochromocytomas are derived from APUD[4] cells of the neural crest.

The tumors appear not to be congenitally associated with cyanosis; the soonest they are seen is in early adolescence.

(1) Circulation. **29**: 750-757 (1964). Seven cases of pheochromocytoma.
(2) Am J Dis Child. **112**: 251-255 (1966). One case of a pheochromocytoma.
(3) Johns Hopkins Med J. **142**: 18-21 (1978). One case of a chemodectoma.
(4) The confusing taxonomy of cells and tumors derived from neural crest cells is admirably described in: Hosp Practice. **10(10)**: 117-126 (1975). APUD stands for "amine precursor uptake decarboxylation."

---

* *paroxysmal atrial tachyarrhythmia*

Surprisingly, polyuria occurs in roughly 50% of patients with a paroxysmal atrial tachyarrhythmia (including fib, flutter, PAT, and WPW);[1,2] why it is so underreported to physicians is unclear.[2] Polyuria after nodal[3] or ventricular[1] tachycardia is rare.

The polyuria can be voluminous (1.8 liters in one case[4]), but does not occur with paroxysms of less than 20 minutes or with heart rates less than 110/min.[1,3] Onset is 20 to 30 minutes after the attack begins, but can start as late as 60 min. It may last as long as 8 hours if the tachycardia lasts that long.[1] Urination occurs as often as every 10 minutes early in the diuresis,[2] leading to interesting anecdotes.[1,2]

Syncope (not uncommon), angina, and right-sided congestive heart failure do not inhibit the polyuria; with acute left ventricular failure, the diuresis is prevented, but may follow the termination of the attack as the patient recovers from heart failure.[1,3]

The pathogenesis of the phenomenon was obscure[3] until elevated levels of atrial natriuretic factor (ANF) were found in post-tachycardic patients.[4,5]

Roughly 30% of migraine patients have polyuria during an attack, commonly as the headache subsides.[6]

(1) Br Heart J. **25**: 273-282 (1963). Posthumous clinical description by Paul Wood.
(2) Ann Intern Med. **65**: 461-470 (1966). 24 patients.
(3) Br Med J. **289**: 866-868, 1536 (1984). A case of nodal tach polyuria.
(4) New Engl J Med. **312**: 1196-1197 (1985). Lancet. **I**: 1211 only (1985). Levels of ANF.
(5) J Am Coll Cardiol. **9**: 509-514 (1987). ANF in atrial tachyarrhythmias.
(6) Arch Neurol. **15**: 356-361 (1966). Lacks further details.
(–) New Engl J Med. **315**: 1398-1401 (1986). Atrial endocrine function in artificial heart patients.

---

* *most severe degree of pulmonary edema*

A letter to the *Annals*[1] reported that the distribution of sweat in 48 patients with pulmonary edema seemed to correlate with the severity of the condition. Sweat only on the forehead correlated with the mildest degree of pulmonary edema, sweat on the forehead and chest with an intermediate degree, and sweat on the forehead and chest and abdomen with the most severe degree. Furthermore, changes in the sweat pattern (either receding or progressing) were indicative of changes in the degree of pulmonary edema.

(1) Ann Intern Med. **101**: 402 only (1984). Letter.
(–) Ann Intern Med. **99**: 808-822 (1983). Review of pulmonary edema.

Heart HE-006

Young man in vigorous good health
with
right ventricular dilatation on echocardiogram

Heart HE-007

Elderly patient in the coronary care unit,
not on lidocaine or an H_2 blocker,
with an acute change in mental status

Heart HE-008

Patient with endocarditis
who has an embolic occlusion of a large artery

** patient is a fighter pilot*[1]

This association probably results from the cardiovascular response to the sustained acceleration forces (G forces) typically encountered in modern high performance jet aircraft. In reference 1, a baboon was catheterized, placed in a centrifuge, accelerated to $+7\ G_Z$ (that is, seven gravities pulling blood inferiorly out of the head), and kept at $+7\ G_Z$ for 23 seconds. Systolic LV pressures rose from 116 (resting) to 150 torr (at the end of the high-G run). RV systolic pressures, however, went from 18 (resting) to 70 (midway through the run) to 120 torr (at end).

A slightly different medical aspect of flying high performance aircraft has attracted a good deal of scientific interest: Do pilots father a disproportionately higher number of daughters than sons? Study results have been conflicting.[2,3,4] Men in other professions (anesthesiology,[3] diving[5]) have been reported to be girl-fathers. Illness (for example, multiple sclerosis,[6] lymphoma,[7] hepatitis B[8]), birth order, sex of previous offspring, season, rainfall, and war may also affect the sex ratio of offspring.[4]

(1) Aviation Space Env Med. **57**: A11 (1986). Abstract number 59 presented at the 1986 Aerospace Medical Association meeting. No description of the time course was provided.
(2) Human Biol. **33**: 1-10 (1961). 59 girls vs 35 boys born to fathers who recently flew fighters.
(3) Aviat Space Env Med. **47**: 889-892 (1976). Effects of stress on sex ratio of offspring.
(4) Aviat Space Env Med. **58**: 707-709 (1987). Retrospective study supports girl-fathering tendency.
(5) Lancet. **II**: 152 only (1982). Letter about Australian abalone divers.
(6) New Engl J Med. **305**: 1157 only (1981). Multiple sclerosis.
(7) New Engl J Med. **306**: 367-368 (1982). Lymphoma.
(8) Science. **201**: 687-692 (1978). Also notes effects of blood group.

** ethanol intoxication*[1,2,3]
** Wernicke encephalopathy*[4]

Nitroglycerin (TNG) is relatively insoluble in water, thus most commercial preparations of parenteral TNG use ethanol and propylene glycol as diluents.[5] Continuous infusion of high dose TNG (range, 1250 to 2470 mcg/min) in four elderly patients resulted in ethanol intoxication associated with serum levels of 21 to 178 mg/dL and the smell of alcohol on the breath.[1,2,3]

Some of these patients later gave a history of lifelong sensitivity to alcohol, but in one case the patient received the equivalent of 48 mL of 86 proof whiskey per hour! From 0.06 to 0.14 mL of ethanol is delivered per milligram of TNG.[2]

A nonalcoholic 74-year-old man became obtunded (and lost his corneal and caloric reflexes!) after 2 days of high dose (1250 mcg/min) TNG infusion. Serum ethanol was 21 mg/dL. He recovered completely after the TNG was discontinued and thiamine administered. Re-institution of TNG for recurrent chest pain produced identical neurologic abnormalities that again responded to thiamine.[4] There is little doubt this was Wernicke encephalopathy, but the biochemical trigger is unclear.[5]

(1) New Engl J Med. **310**: 1123 only (1984). A 73-year-old man.
(2) Ann Intern Med. **101**: 498-499 (1984). Two cases.
(3) Ann Intern Med. **102**: 274 only (1985). A 69-year-old man.
(4) Ann Intern Med. **101**: 500 only (1984). Case of Wernicke encephalopathy.
(5) Ann Intern Med. **102**: 134 only (1985). Two letters: Wernicke rejoinder & formulary change.
(–) Intravenous TNG may precipitate acute gouty arthritis [Arch Intern Med. **148**: 1505-2506 (1988).].

** fungal endocarditis*
** nonbacterial thrombotic endocarditis (NBTE)*
** atrial myxoma*

Large, friable vegetations are characteristic of these diseases. Embolic occlusion of a large blood vessel (such as the femoral artery) is uncommon in bacterial endocarditis, and should alert the physician to the possibility of the above disorders.[1] *Staphylococcus aureus* vegetations are "occasionally" big enough to occlude a large vessel,[2] but it would not be surprising if, someday, bacterial vegetations in patients infected with the human immunodeficiency virus are shown to routinely be of sufficient size to do likewise.[3]

NBTE may occur not only with carcinoma (especially mucin-secreting adenocarcinoma), but also in nonmalignant disorders such as congestive heart failure, pneumonia, pyelonephritis, and glomerulonephritis.[4]

(1) New Engl J Med. **291**: 1122-1126 (1974). Classic review of endocarditis.
(2) "Infective endocarditis." AW Karchmer & MN Swartz. In: Scientific American Medicine. E Rubenstein & DD Federman (eds). New York: Scientific American (9/88). 7:XVIII:4-5.
(3) In a study that did not consider HIV status, 60% of intravenous drug users with right-sided endocarditis had large (at least 1 cm) tricuspid vegetations. 60% of these were due to S. Aureus [Arch Intern Med. **148**: 2461-2465 (1988).].
(4) Ann Intern Med. **46**: 255-273 (1957). 78 cases of NBTE.

Heart HE-009

A patient two weeks after a myocardial infarction,
on a normal dose of quinidine,
without clinical or electrocardiographic signs of toxicity,
but with serum drug level of 11 mg%

Heart HE-010

Man with a heart murmur,
poised to jump out the window

Heart HE-011

Chest pain so bad you're afraid you're going to live

(as opposed to chest pain so bad you're afraid you're going to die)

** high alpha-1-acid glycoprotein level; normal therapeutic level of free quinidine*[1]

Normally, 90% of the quinidine in the bloodstream is bound to protein. In contrast to acidic drugs, which bind mainly to serum albumin, basic drugs such as quinidine may bind more avidly to other serum proteins. Thus, quinidine, like lidocaine, disopyramide, propranolol, and imipramine, preferentially binds to a protein called alpha-1-acid glycoprotein, which also happens to be an acute phase reactant.

It is well known that the physiologic stress of myocardial infarction (MI) will elevate the concentration of acute phase reactants; after an MI, the alpha-1-acid glycoprotein level increases as early as the second post-infarction day, and remains elevated for 3 to 8 (or more) weeks.

The usual therapeutic range of serum quinidine levels is 2 to 6 mg%. The elevated serum quinidine concentration in the patient reported resulted from a combination of a near tripling of the alpha-1-acid glycoprotein level and an increase in the fraction of all serum quinidine bound to protein (to 97%). The level of free (that is, non-protein-bound) quinidine was 0.35 mg% (usual, 0.2 to 0.6). The absence of signs of quinidine toxicity in this patient supports the hypothesis that the concentration of unbound drug determines the intensity of quinidine's effect.

(1) Ann Intern Med. **107**: 48-50 (1987). Case report and nice discussion.
(–) Circulation. **70**: 472-478 (1984). Varied binding of anti-arrhythmics during MI evolution.

** aortic regurgitation*[1]

[This is clearly the most bizarre of the numerous peripheral manifestations of aortic regurgitation (less properly known as "aortic incompetency"), but if you can't trust Osler, who can you trust?[2]]

"Here may appropriately be mentioned the connection between mental symptoms and cardiac disease, as they are oftenest seen with [aortic incompetency]. An admirable account of the relations between insanity and disease of the heart is found in Mickle's Gulstonian lectures for 1888. In general medical practice we seldom find marked mental symptoms, except toward the close of the disease, when there may be delirium, hallucinations, and morbid impulses. It is to be remembered that in many heart cases this terminal delirium is uræmic. The irritability and peevishness sometimes found in persons the subject of organic heart-disease cannot, I think, be associated with it in any special manner. We do meet insanity, breaking out in patients with aortic and mitral disease, in the stage of compensation, which appears to be related definitely to the cardiac lesion. It is important to bear this in mind, for cases occasionally display suicidal tendencies. I have twice had patients throw themselves from the window of the ward."[1]

(1) The Principles and Practice of Medicine. W Osler. New York: Appleton (1892) p 607.
(2) Certainly not Egerton Y. Davis (card NO-001).

(Trunkey distinction[1])

** pain of aortic dissection (as opposed to the pain of myocardial infarction)*

The pain of aortic dissection (AD), which is absent or minimal in 10% to 15% of cases,[2,3] is usually "the most severe, agonizing, excruciating, or intense" pain the patient has ever experienced.[2] Words like ripping, tearing, and choking are used to describe it.[2,3] Characteristically, the patient is restless and moves about, vainly trying to find a position to relieve the pain.[4] (This is in marked distinction to patients with myocardial infarction, who typically lie very quietly, scarcely moving, with "no inclination to groan or cry out."[5]) Morphine doses much larger than those commonly used in myocardial infarction (MI) may be necessary for relief. The initial pain may occur anywhere from the ears to the legs, but is in the chest in 80% of cases.[2] Its location may sometimes be used to predict the dissection site, but a more important clue distinguishing AD from MI is the migratory nature of the pain as the dissection advances through the aorta.[2,3,4]

Curiously, over half of AD patients who have clinical signs of shock will have systolic blood pressures above 100 mm Hg. (It is thought that pre-existing hypertension may be responsible for this phenomenon.)[2] Occlusion of one or both subclavian arteries can also lead to an incorrect diagnosis of systemic hypotension.[3]

(1) D Trunkey MD, who heard it from a patient. UCSF, circa 1972. [Mis-attributed in 1st printing.]
(2) Medicine. **37**: 217-279 (1958). Fabulous review of 505 cases. Better control of hypertension may have altered some of the aspects of the disease since 1958, and, hence, some of the statistics.
(3) New Engl J Med. **317**: 1060-1067 (1987). Recent review. See also cards NC-001 & TH-009.
(4) Heart Disease. 3rd ed. E Braunwald (ed). Philadelphia: Saunders (1988). p 1235.
(5) Ibid. p 1555. Vivid first-person account of myocardial infarction.
(–) Aortic dissection may elevate creatine phosphokinase [Arch Intern Med. **148**: 2184-2186 (1988).].

Heart - Auscultation HE-301

Noise heard with the unaided ear at a distance from the chest,
synchronous with the heart beat

Heart - Auscultation HE-302

Clearly perceived diastolic murmur,
closely approximating a pure musical tone
or the coo of a dove

Heart - Auscultation HE-303

Diastolic murmur of aortic regurgitation,
radiating down the right side of the sternum

According to Bean,[1] the causes of these noises may be classified as follows:

35% – heart murmurs (due to valve rupture [esp. aortic] or other lesion)
21% – interstitial mediastinal or pulmonary emphysema (such as a loud Hamman sign)
16% – pneumothorax (spontaneous or traumatic)
15% – pneumopericardium
5% – heart percussing an air-filled colon or esophagus ("ectopic borborygmi")
4% – pulmonary air embolism
4% – miscellaneous

These data are from 1953; since then prosthetic heart valves have presumably become the most common cause. The loudest sound described in the series emanated from a man with "rupture of a heart valve," and "could be heard in the room below."

Ironically, on his deathbed, Laennec, the inventor of the stethoscope, developed such a distantly heard heart sound.

(1) J Am Med Assn. **152**: 1293-1301 (1953). No bibliography. An expanded version with references is: Monographs in Medicine, Series I. WB Bean (ed). Baltimore: Williams & Wilkins (1952). pp 22-65.
(–) For more on "noises heard at a distance from the chest," see: [a] Rare Diseases and Lesions. WB Bean. Springfield, IL: Thomas (1967). pp 134-137; and [b] Ann Intern Med. **42**: 1214-1226 (1955).

(dove-coo murmur[1])

* *aortic regurgitation (AR)*

This murmur often has a phenomenal degree of audibility; it may be heard on the top of the head, in the extremities, or without a stethoscope (card HE-301). In most cases, pathologic studies have shown eversion, perforation, or laceration along the margin of an aortic valve cusp or along the line of attachment of a cusp.

The murmur has also been described as similar to a "sea-gull cry," "humming top," or "whistling."

Despite the audibility of this murmur, the typical AR murmur can be difficult to hear. One study found that the ward physicians (that is, the housestaff) missed 53% of the AR murmurs in their patients.[2]

(1) Ann Intern Med. **42**: 1214-1226 (1955). Dove-coo murmur.
(2) Am Heart J. **71**: 627-634 (1966). Aortic regurgitation in the elderly.

(Harvey sign)

* *aortic regurgitation caused by disease external to the valve (that is, dilatation and rightward displacement of the aortic root[1,2])*

* *can also occur with deformity limited to the valve, or with rightward displacement of the heart*

In 95% of rheumatic aortic regurgitation (AR) the murmur is louder in the left third intercostal space than in the right. When the murmur is louder on the right, another cause is suggested, namely one associated with aortic root disease: aortic aneurysm, sinus of Valsalva aneurysm, syphilis, the Marfan syndrome, osteogenesis imperfecta, rheumatoid spondylitis, medionecrosis, trauma, hypertension, aortitis, and arteriosclerosis.

Of course, just as the conditions above may sometimes have AR murmurs that are louder on the left side of the sternum, diseases limited to the aortic valve may sometimes produce murmurs louder to the right of the sternum than the left (for example, bacterial endocarditis, syphilis, trauma, ventricular septal defect, sclerotic changes).

(1) Am J Med Sci. **245**: 533-543 (1963). Original description. Note that in 1963 80% of aortic regurgitation was the result of rheumatic fever.
(2) Cardiac Diagnosis and Treatment. 3rd ed. NO Fowler. Hagerstown, MD: Harper & Row (1980). p 568.
(–) One would expect dextrocardia or pneumothorax to complicate the matter as well.

Heart - Electrocardiogram

HE-601

Flat-line ECG in an alert patient

Heart - Electrocardiogram

HE-602

In a patient with chest pain,
ECG shows loss of anterior wall voltage when supine,
but is normal when patient sits or stands

Heart - Electrocardiogram

HE-603

Technically accurate, but markedly abnormal ECG
that normalizes when the limb electrodes are switched
to opposite sides

** artificial heart*[1]

Dr. Barney Clark's postoperative electrocardiogram was without electrical activity. The Utah total artificial heart is powered pneumatically.[1] A later article, however, notes that the patient's natural atria are not removed during surgery, and that P waves are visible on postoperative ECGs.[2]

Patients who undergo conventional ("orthotopic") heart transplants usually retain their native atria as well.[3] Because the donor heart is implanted with both of its atria, the post-transplant ECG may have two independent streams of P waves, only one of which is coupled to QRS complexes.[4,5] Interestingly, P waves sensed in the native atria have been used to pace the donated atria, thereby providing functional chronotropic innervation to the biologically denervated donor heart.[6]

Marginally relevant to this discussion is the claim of Paul Dudley White that, in the presence of ventricular standstill, atrial contractions can be auscultated.[7]

(1) New Engl J Med. **310**: 273-278 (1984). Pre- and postoperative ECGs are on page 274.
(2) New Engl J Med. **315**: 1398-1401 (1986). Atrial endocrine function in artificial heart patients.
(3) Surg Clin North Am. **66**: 477-489 (1986). Transplantation technique.
(4) Hosp Practice. **23(11)**: 37, 40, 42 (1988). ECGs in heart transplant patients.
(5) Rarely, there will be a transplant in which the native heart is not removed. Without this knowledge, attempted interpretation of post-operative ECGs involves prolonged head-scratching.
(6) J Heart Transplant. **7**: 23-25 (1988). Pacemakers in heart transplant patients.
(7) Clues in the Diagnosis and Treatment of Heart Disease. 2nd ed. PD White. Springfield, IL: Thomas (1956). p 55.
(–) JAMA. **259**: 849-859 (1988). Report of four patients with an artificial heart.

** left pneumothorax*[1]

The specific ECG changes seen in left pneumothorax include: (1) progressive voltage loss in the precordial leads, sometimes with near-complete loss of R waves from V_1 to V_6, (2) right axis deviation, and (3) nonspecific precordial T wave flattening and sometimes T wave inversion.

The changes are caused by three factors: (1) movement of the heart (and mediastinum) to the right and therefore away from the precordial leads, (2) air interposed between the heart and the chest leads, and (3) some degree of anatomic clockwise rotation of the heart.

Because these patients have chest pain, the ECG may mistakenly support the diagnosis of an anterolateral myocardial infarction. Normalization of the precordial ECG pattern when the patient sits up or stands is said to be pathognomonic of left pneumothorax.[1]

In cases of right pneumothorax, the mediastinum is shifted to the left, and the pattern of decreased precordial voltage is not seen.[1] Spontaneous pneumothorax may also produce the ECG pattern of acute cor pulmonale (that is, P-pulmonale in II, III, F, V_1; an $S_1Q_3T_3$ pattern; and an rsR′ in V_1).[3]

(1) Myocardial Infarction: Electrocardiographic Differential Diagnosis. 2nd ed. AL Goldberger. St. Louis: Mosby (1979). pp 39-41. Copiously referenced.
(2) Ann Intern Med. **80**: 375-379 (1974). Nice summary of ECG changes in left pneumothorax.
(3) The Electrocardiogram and Chest X-Ray in the Diseases of the Heart. AM Master et al. Philadelphia: Lea & Febiger (1963). pp 329-331.

** dextrocardia*

Of course, this maneuver will only normalize the limb lead tracings; recording right chest leads (V_{1R} to V_{6R}) will normalize the precordial pattern as well. Correcting the ECG in this manner permits more rapid identification of underlying ECG abnormalities.

A standard "left-sided" ECG in a patient with dextrocardia shows poor R wave progression and progressive loss of voltage. QS waves are usually seen in the left precordial leads and in leads I and aVL. In fact, aVL and aVR both have their usual tracings inverted.

The Electrocardiogram and Chest X-Ray in the Diseases of the Heart. AM Master et al. Philadelphia: Lea & Febiger (1963).
Myocardial Infarction: Electrocardiographic Differential Diagnosis. 2nd ed. AL Goldberger. St. Louis: Mosby (1979). p 39. Copiously referenced.

Heart - Electrocardiogram

HE-604

Decrease of the PR interval over several years

Immunology / Infection

IM-001

Rubor et tumor cum calore et dolore

Immunology / Infection

IM-002

Syndrome of an upper respiratory infection in a welder

* *Fabry disease*[1]

The multisystem pathology of Fabry disease results from accumulation of glycolipid in body tissues (card AB-004), including the heart. Cardiovascular disease occurs in most hemizygotic males, commonly manifest as ischemic heart disease, congestive heart failure, or cardiomegaly. Mitral regurgitation and aortic stenosis are the most frequent valvular lesions. Systemic hypertension may result from renal disease.[2]

An abbreviated PR interval has been reported several times in Fabry disease.[2] In two patients followed for 10 years, serial electrocardiograms documented a decrease in the PR interval (from 0.18 to 0.11 seconds in one, and 0.12 to 0.10 in the other). The authors hypothesized that glycolipid deposition in the atrioventricular junction was responsible for accelerating conduction.[1]

Other conditions, such as chronic lung disease, acute myocardial infarction, ectopic impulse formation, enhanced sympathetic tone (including that seen in pheochromocytoma[3]), Cushing disease, hyperthyroidism, and Pompe disease (a glycogen storage disorder), have also been associated with short PR intervals. The Lown-Ganong-Levine syndrome is a short PR interval plus normal QRS complexes plus paroxysmal rapid heart action.[3]

(1) Angiology. **29**: 562-568 (1978). Case reports.
(2) The Metabolic Basis of Inherited Disease. 5th ed. JB Stanbury et al (eds). New York: McGraw-Hill (1983). pp 906-944. Complete review of Fabry disease.
(3) J Am Coll Cardiol. **3**: 872-875 (1984). Removing the pheo returned the PR to normal.

---

* *acute inflammation*[1]

[Apologies for this card, but the author has found this ancient dictum so useful in clinical practice that he feels compelled to include it.]

The four cardinal signs of acute inflammation were set forth by Aurelius Cornelius Celsus, a Roman who lived in the reign of Tiberius Cæsar. He was "not a physician, but a private gentleman [who] compiled or, more probably, translated encyclopedic treatises on medicine, agriculture, and other subjects."[2]

The fifth cardinal sign of inflammation, loss of function (*functio læsa*), was promulgated by Rudolf Virchow in 1858,[1] and not by Galen as has long been taught.[3]

(1) The Healing Hand. G Majno. Cambridge, MA: Harvard (1975). pp 370-374, 412-413. Discusses the birth of the four cardinal signs and the discoverer of the fifth sign.
(2) History of Medicine. 4th ed. FH Garrison. Philadelphia: Saunders (1929). pp 107-109.
(3) Bull NY Acad Med. **47**: 303-323 (1971). Seeks the discoverer of the fifth sign.

---

* *metal fume fever (MFF)*[1,2]

Exposure to metal fumes (usually Zn, Cu, or Mg, but also Al, Sb, Fe, Mn, and Ni) can produce a syndrome very much like a viral infection: fever (38.8 to 40.0°C), malaise, arthralgia, cough, sore throat, and chest tightness that last 1 to 2 days. The chest x-ray is usually normal and a mild leukocytosis is common. Symptoms develop 4 to 12 hours after exposure, hampering diagnosis.

Re-exposure within 1 to 2 days does not cause recurrent symptoms, but later exposures may. Thus, metal fume fever is more likely to occur after several days away from work, and is known as Monday fever by some workers.

Metal fume fever has no known long-term adverse effects, but life-threatening chemical pneumonitis can develop in industrial workers after similar exposures and with similar initial symptoms.[1,2,3] For example, cadmium, which is present in some hobby shop solder,[2] is especially dangerous. (The use of cadmium oxide as an agent of chemical warfare has been considered.[1]) After an MFF-like prodrome, pulmonary edema follows, usually within 24 hours of exposure. After 72 hours this resolves and a proliferative interstitial pneumonitis sets in that can progress to alveolar obliteration and fibrosis. The fatality rate is 15% to 20%, usually within 7 days.[1] Do not rely on history: Patients are often unaware they work with cadmium-containing products.[3]

(1) Occupational Lung Disorders. 2nd ed. WR Parkes. London: Butterworths (1982). pp 454-463.
(2) USAF Aerospace Medicine Primary Course. Brooks AFB, TX. 26 Feb 1985.
(3) Chest. **86**: 789-791 (1984). Similarity of cadmium pneumonitis and metal fume fever.
(–) Morb Mort Weekly Report. **36**: 515-516, 521-522 (1987). A related illness: polymer fume fever.

Immunology / Infection IM-003

Anaphylaxis after touching another person

Immunology / Infection IM-004

Streptococcus bovis bacteremia

Immunology / Infection IM-005

History of
two episodes of disseminated Neisserial infection

** reaction to mosquito repellent*

"A 42-year-old woman with no prior atopic history touched a companion who had just sprayed himself with an insect repellent containing 52 percent deet. Generalized pruritus rapidly developed and progressed to generalized angioedema. The woman was rushed to an emergency room, becoming nauseated en route and losing consciousness. On arrival her blood pressure was 70/40 mm Hg. The patient responded to treatment with parenteral epinephrine, diphenhydramine, and corticosteroids." Controlled re-challenge a week later also provoked severe symptoms.[1]

Deet (N,N-diethyl-m-toluamide) is found in commercial products like *Off!* and *6-12 Plus* insect repellents. About 10% to 15% of each dose is systemically absorbed through the skin. Toxic encephalopathy, sometimes fatal, has been reported in children sprayed repeatedly with deet. Local allergic reactions (such as contact urticaria) and toxic reactions (*eg*, erythema, burning, and blistering) also occur.[2]

Life-threatening anaphylaxis has followed the use of topical bacitracin and neomycin ointments as well.[3] "It is thus important for clinicians to consider topical preparations when they evaluate a case of anaphylaxis of unknown origin."[1]

(1) New Engl J Med. **307**: 1341-1342 (1982). Letter.
(2) Med Lett Drugs Ther. **27**: 62-64 (1985). Insect repellents.
(3) Arch Dermatol. **120**: 909-911 (1984). Anaphylaxis to topical agents. See card GU-004.

** colonic neoplasm or other gastrointestinal malignancy*[1]
** benign conditions associated with lost bowel-wall integrity*[2]

Often classified in the past as an enterococcus or as a viridans Streptococcus by clinical microbiologic laboratories, *S. bovis* attained recognition as a frequent cause of infective endocarditis once appropriate tests on blood culture isolates began.[3] Later, it was recognized that *S. bovis* endocarditis was associated with carcinoma of the colon and, further, that 56% of colon cancer patients carried the organism in their gut, *vs* 10% to 16% of normal controls.[4] Finally, in a series of 15 patients with *S. bovis* bacteremia who underwent a complete gastrointestinal evaluation including colonoscopy, surgery, or autopsy, neoplasms were discovered in 13.[5,6]

S. bovis bacteremia has been seen with other GI neoplasms.[1,5,7] Thus, calls have been made for all patients with *S. bovis* bacteremia to undergo aggressive GI, especially colonic, evaluation.[5] However, the many benign conditions also co-reported[2] suggest that *S. bovis* bacteremia may only be a marker of decreased bowel wall integrity.[7]

(1) Carcinomas: stomach, pancreas, mouth; lymphomas: colon, stomach; sarcomas: gastric Kaposi.
(2) Diverticulosis, rectal manipulation, rectal volvulus, perirectal abscess, colonic ulceration, radiation entercolitis, hemorrhoids.
(3) Am J Med. **57**: 239-250 (1974). Enterococcal vs S. bovis endocarditis.
(4) New Engl J Med. **297**: 800-802 (1977). Patients in this report are used in reference 5, too.
(5) Ann Intern Med. **91**: 560-562 (1979). Weak study: no controls, re-uses data of reference 4.
(6) 2 patients had colonic adenocarcinomas; 5, villous adenomas with carcinomas; 1, a colonic adenomatous polyp with carcinoma; 3, colonic adenomatous polyp(s); and 2, esophageal carcinomas.
(7) New Engl J Med. **316**: 529-540 (1987). CPC, with a two paragraph discussion of S. bovis.

** complement deficiency*

Complement factor C3, once activated by either the classical pathway (factors C1, C4, C2) or the alternative pathway (factors D, P, B), normally triggers the bactericidal arm of the cascade (factors C5 to C9). Although a homozygous deficiency of any complement factor[1] predisposes to severe pyogenic infections, a homozygous "late" defect (C5-C9) is associated with systemic neisserial infection to the near exclusion of other pathogens.[2,3]

Ten to fifteen percent of patients with meningococcal meningitis (MM) or disseminated gonorrhea (*eg*, arthralgia or dermatitis) have an inherited complement deficiency; 45% of this 10% to 15% will later have at least one recurrence of systemic neisserial infection.[2]

Management of these patients is unclear, as MM in them is typically *less* severe than in normals.[2] There is an exception, however: Properdin deficiency (McKusick 31206) is an X-linked disorder of the alternate pathway that predisposes to fulminant, fatal MM. Unfortunately, and unlike the CH_{50} assay for the combined activity of factors C1-C9, assays for alternative pathway activity are not generally available. Nevertheless, a family history of fulminant meningococcal disease restricted to males should provoke testing of the alternative pathway: Evidence suggests that meningococcal vaccine offers some protection to properdin-deficient males.[4]

(1) Except for properdin, complement proteins are autosomally inherited (reference 4).
(2) Medicine. **63**: 243-273 (1983). Definitive review of infection and complement deficiency.
(3) Deficiency of classical pathway factors or of C3, whether heterozygous or homozygous, generally predisposes to autoimmune/collagen-vascular disease (reference 2).
(4) New Engl J Med. **316**: 922-926 (1987). Properdin deficiency and fatal meningococcemia.
(–) Other immunopathies are linked to meningococcal disease [Arch Intern Med. **148**: 754 only (1988).].

Lung LU-001

Heme negative "hemoptysis"

Lung LU-002

Chronic sino-pulmonary infections and male infertility

Lung LU-003

Childhood ability to hold breath or swim underwater much longer than others

(pseudohemoptysis)

* *pulmonary infection with* Serratia marcesans[1]

This gram-negative rod produces a red pigment that has been masquerading as blood since at least the 6th century BC, when Pythagorus noticed a bloody discoloration on foodstuffs.[1]

Other causes of pseudohemoptysis certainly exist, as in the workmen of a 19th century brick and tile factory who noticed "bloody-looking sputa ... during the days on which they were employed in emptying the kilns of their burnt and dry contents."[2] Rifampin may impart an orange-red color to sputum, saliva, urine, feces, tears, and sweat; patients should so be warned.[3]

(1) New Engl J Med. **300**: 867-893 (1979). Clinical review, as well as more of this bug's fascinating history.
(2) Sputum: Its Microscopy and Diagnostic and Prognostic Significances. F Troup. Edinburgh: Oliver & Boyd (1886). p 218.
(3) Goodman & Gilman's The Pharmacological Basis of Therapeutics. 6th ed. AG Gilman et al (eds). New York: Macmillan (1980). p 1204.

---

* *Young syndrome*[1]
* *cystic fibrosis*
* *immotile cilia syndrome*

Men with Young syndrome "have only mildly impaired respiratory function and normal spermatogenesis; the azoospermia is due to obstruction of the epididymis by inspissated secretions." The sperm appear normal, and there are no ultrastructural cilial disorders. Some patients have fathered children before presentation, suggesting a progressive increase in the degree of obstruction. Furthermore, it appears that restoration of fertility is possible in some cases.[1]

The sinopulmonary infections are mild, have onset in early childhood, and generally improve after adolescence. Deficiencies of immunoglobulins or alpha$_1$ antitrypsin also cause chronic sinopulmonary infection.[1]

Young syndrome is probably as common as Klinefelter syndrome, and appears to be autosomal recessive. Sweat and pancreatic function are normal in patients with the Young syndrome.[1] The Kartagener syndrome seems to be a subgroup of the immotile cilia syndrome rather than identical with it.[2]

(1) New Engl J Med. **310**: 3-9 (1984). Young syndrome. McKusick 27900.
(2) Am Rev Respir Dis. **124**: 107-109 (1981). Editorial on aspects of ciliary dysfunction.
(-) Inherited Diseases of the Lung. J Lieberman. Philadelphia: Saunders (1988). See pp 87-98. Emphasizes value of the reproductive history in male patients with chronic bronchitis.

---

* *predisposes to blue bloater type of chronic obstructive pulmonary disease*

As chronic airways obstruction progresses, especially without vigorous treatment, the clinical picture tends to diverge into a spectrum of symptoms, the two extremes of which are easily identified as the pink puffer and blue bloater.

"It is hypothesized that the dyspneic-cachectic or pink puffer syndrome occurs in persons whose ventilatory and perfusing capacities are lost at approximately the same rate.... The cardiac-polycythemic or blue bloater picture, on the other hand, occurs in subjects who develop diffuse ventilatory obstruction before they lose their parenchymal vasculature and their capacity to circulate blood and perfuse gases; in other words, they have chronic bronchial and bronchiolar inflammation with only mild or no destructive emphysema, with resultant marked ventilation/ perfusion inequality."

To develop the blue bloater condition seems to require "subjects whose respiratory centers are hyporesponsive to changes in pO_2 (and pCO_2 and pH, too, in all probability) on either an acquired or a genetic basis. In support of a possible genetic basis, some of these patients recall in their youth being able to swim under water and hold their breath much longer than others, long before the onset of any indication of cardiopulmonary disease."

Textbook of Pulmonary Diseases. 2nd ed. GL Baum (ed). Boston: Little Brown (1974). pp 586-587.

Lung LU-004

Pseudomonas bronchitis in a young adult

Lung LU-005

More than 10% eosinophils in the leukocyte differential count of a pleural effusion

Lung LU-006

Copious sputum, settling into three layers

* *cystic fibrosis (CF)*

Even in patients with hypogammaglobulinemia or defective neutrophil function, *Pseudomonas aeruginosa* is an unlikely pathogen. For reasons unknown, "patients with cystic fibrosis have a unique susceptibility to developing chronic *P. aeruginosa* bronchitis. ... Adult patients with chronic or recurrent respiratory infections, in whom *P. aeruginosa* is isolated from the sputum, should be suspected of having late-onset CF" and should have a sweat chloride test.[1]

In general, the sweat-chloride test retains its diagnostic value even in older CF patients.[2] However, a variant/subtype of CF, characterized by chronic Pseudomonas bronchitis and absence of digestive symptoms has been identified in which sweat chloride tests yield intermediate values.[3]

(1) Medical Knowledge Self-Assessment Program VII. Philadelphia: American College of Physicians (1985). p 21 & (Book B1) p 3.
(2) The Metabolic Basis of Inherited Disease. 5th ed. JB Stanbury et al (eds). New York: McGraw-Hill (1983). pp 1896-1897.
(3) JAMA. **239**: 2676-2680 (1978). CF variant.
(–) Thorax. **42**: 526-532 (1987). CF in adolescents and adults.

---

* *nontuberculous, nonmalignant cause*[1]

Although different authors have variously required that 5, 10, 20, or even 50% of all cells in a pleural effusion be eosinophils before the effusion can be labelled "eosinophilic," 10% is the most common value used.[1] Depending on this cutoff value, from 3% to 10% of pleural effusions are eosinophilic. (Note that the percentage of eosinophils taken into consideration should be that found in the first pleural aspirate; pleural taps can themselves increase the number of eosinophils).[1]

Roughly 50 causes of eosinophilic pleural effusions (EPEs) have been reported, including infection (bacterial, viral, fungal, parasitic), hypersensitivity states, trauma, malignancy, and connective tissue diseases.[1] Blood eosinophilia is a frequent accompaniment, except in cases of pneumonia, pulmonary infarction, carcinoma, or trauma.[1] Some authors claim that pleural fluid eosinophilia is of little use in the differential diagnosis of pleural effusions, but recent studies have shown that the likelihoods of malignancy and tuberculosis are considerably reduced when EPEs are present.[2,3] Furthermore, when associated with pneumonia, EPEs signify a good prognosis; they are said to virtually never become infected.[1,4]

(1) Pleural Effusion. AO Vladutiu. Mt. Kisco, NY: Futura (1986). pp 306-313.
(2) Am J Med. **77**: 915-920 (1984). Analysis using Bayes' rule.
(3) Acta Med Scand. **210**: 129-135 (1981). Total and differential white counts in pleural effusions.
(4) Med Clin N Am. **61**: 1339-1352 (1977). Does not cite data to support the claim.

---

* *bronchiectasis*[1]
* *lung abscess*[2] *(?)*
* *chronic bronchitis*[1]

This "classical" sign of bronchiectasis, mentioned but fleetingly in modern texts,[2,3] and said not to be "often encountered,"[2] is detailed in Troup's century-old monograph: "After standing undisturbed... for hours or days [the sputum] separates into three layers; the undermost and heaviest consists of the sputa proper, and contains a relatively large amount of unaltered pus-cells; the middle is a turbid, glutinous, yellow-green liquid with ragged flocci of mucus suspended in it; the uppermost is a... semi-transparent or dirty brown or red fluid turbidity."[1] The sputum of chronic bronchitis, after standing for "many days," is similar, except the topmost layer is a "large-bubbled persistent covering of saliva, or a foul sloppy serosity in which molecular debris, fatty disintegrated and disintegrating cells and epithelium are abundant."[1]

Tri-layered sputum is supposedly "classical" for lung abscess as well, but the only written account I've found describes *four* layers in the sputum of Staphylococcal lung abscess.[2]

(1) Sputum: Its Microscopy and Diagnostic and Prognostic Significances. Francis Troup. Edinburgh: Oliver and Boyd (1886). pp 188-189, 193-194. Is this the sign's original description?
(2) Pulmonary Diseases and Disorders. AP Fishman. New York: McGraw-Hill (1980). pp 103, 1053, 1215.
(3) Textbook of Pulmonary Diseases. 3rd ed. GL Baum & E Wolinsky. Boston: Little, Brown (1983). p 625.

Lung LU-007

Dyspnea,
worse when upright than when recumbent

Mouth MO-001

Large, lobulated, orange tonsils

Mouth MO-002

Pain in the angles of the jaw
when chewing solid food

(platypnea)

* *shunting of blood, as seen in pulmonary, cardiac, or hepatic disease*

This symptom requires great care to elicit. A related objective sign is orthodeoxia – arterial oxygen desaturation occurring only in the upright position. Platypnea, which may lurk under the diagnoses 'exertional dyspnea,' 'deconditioning,' or 'functional illness,'[1] can occur by at least three mechanisms:

- *Intrapulmonary shunting.* For example, the pulmonary arteriovenous fistulae of Osler-Weber-Rendu syndrome have a tendency to occur in the lower lobes,[2] resulting in increased shunting of blood through them when the thorax is upright.
- *Intracardiac shunting.* Tilt-table cardiac catheterization has demonstrated that right-to-left shunting through a patent foramen ovale may increase by 3½ times when the upright posture is assumed. The mechanism is unknown. Normal right atrial pressures are the rule, but there is a mysterious tendency for patients with pneumonectomy, pulmonary emboli, or other chronic lung disease to develop these shunts. Surgical closure of the opening may improve symptoms dramatically.[1]
- *An unclear lesion* that is not a pure shunt (because arterial oxygen saturation improves when 100% O_2 is breathed). Typically seen in patients with liver disease, dilated capillaries in the lung bases are thought responsible.[3]

(1) Mayo Clin Proc. **59**: 221-231, 280-281 (1984). 7 platypneic patients; 5 had had pneumonectomy.
(2) Mayo Clin Proc. **58**: 176-181 (1983). Review of pulmonary arteriovenous fistulae.
(3) Mayo Clin Proc. **62**: 164-173 (1987). Interesting discussion of physiology.
(–) Bilateral diaphragmatic paralysis or an intracavitary cardiac mass (eg, ball-valve thrombus) may cause platypnea [Heart Disease. 3rd ed. E Braunwald (ed). Philadelphia: Saunders (1988) pp 3, 1877.], as may severe orthostatic hypotension [in press].

---

* *Tangier disease*[1]

Tangier disease, named after the Chesapeake Bay island home of the two index cases, is an autosomal recessive condition[2] characterized by severe deficiency (or absence) of normal high density lipoprotein (HDL) and by the accumulation of cholesterol esters in bodily tissues. Accumulation of these esters in histiocytes leads to the striking appearance of the tonsils, and to the equally characteristic orange-brown 1- to 2-mm spots studding the rectal mucosa. Liver, spleen, lymph nodes, cornea, heart valves, and other organs may be affected as well. Recurrent "tonsilitis" or symptoms of airway obstruction may lead to tonsilectomy.[1]

Not only HDL, but LDL (low density lipoprotein) is also deficient and abnormal. Total cholesterol levels range from 40 to 125 mg/dL, and may even be under 20. Triglycerides, however, are usually elevated, thereby giving Tangier disease a unique lipid signature among all known diseases. Heterozygotes have normal tonsils and low HDL; like homozygotes, they do not seem at appreciably increased risk for atherosclerotic disease, however, the small number of cases reported makes generalization difficult.[1]

About one third of patients present with symptoms of a peripheral neuropathy,[1] which, in some instances, is clinically similar to syringomyelia.[1,3]

(1) The Metabolic Basis of Inherited Disease. 5th ed. JB Stanbury et al (eds). New York: McGraw-Hill (1983). pp 607-614.
(2) McKusick 20540.
(3) Acta Neurol Scand. **72**: 495-505 (1985). Cites all 33 reported cases of Tangier disease.

(claudication of the jaw[1])

* *giant cell arteritis (GCA)*[2]
* *primary systemic amyloidosis*[3]

Classically considered pathognomonic of GCA, intermittent claudication is an ischemic symptom caused by narrowing or obstruction of the facial branches of the external carotid artery that supply the masticatory muscles. (The facial artery does not develop high-grade atherosclerotic obstruction.) However, a recent study reported jaw claudication in 22 of 193 patients with amyloidosis (9%). Eighteen had amyloid alone and 4 had amyloid associated with myeloma. Typical features of amyloid were present in only half of the 22 cases. Interestingly, 2 also had symptoms of polymyalgia rheumatica.[3]

Ischemic cranial symptoms in GCA are not limited to the jaw or to chewing. Claudication with deglutition, pain in the neck muscles after prolonged speaking, pain in the temporal area with chewing, or pain in the tongue with chewing or talking[2] may occur. Prompt relief of pain with rest distinguishes claudication from temporo-mandibular arthritis and from disorders of the teeth and salivary glands.[2] More unusual symptoms include recurrent choking sensations, talking that precipitates paroxysms of coughing,[4] lancinating pain behind the eyes or ears, and a peculiar deep pain in the throat.[3]

(1) Strictly speaking, "claudication" refers only to symptoms caused by walking [New Engl J Med. **306**: 1297 only (1982).]. Bean has called Takayasu disease "intermittent claudication of the brain" [Rare Diseases and Lesions. WB Bean. Springfield, IL: Thomas (1967). p 45] and, indeed, jaw claudication occurs in this disorder [Acta Med Scand. **149**: 161-178 (1954).].
(2) Medicine. **50**: 1-27 (1971). Classic article on clinical manifestations of GCA.
(3) Medicine. **65**: 173-179 (1986). Study of jaw claudication in amyloidosis.
(4) Ann Intern Med. **101**: 594-597 (1984). Respiratory tract symptoms (cough, sore throat) in GCA.

Mouth MO-003

Linear white grooves
radiating from the corners of the mouth

Mouth MO-004

Multiple blue-black spots on the lips

Mouth - Teeth and Gums MO-701

Notch in biting edge of incisors

(rhagades)

* *stigma of early congenital syphilis*

Congenital syphilis is divided into early and late stages. The early phase occurs between the second and twenty-fifth week of life, and prominently features a skin eruption ("syphilid") most often affecting the chin, circumoral region, palms, soles, and anogenital region.[1] Extreme loss of cutaneous elastic tissue in the circumoral region may occur as a consequence of this eruption, ultimately resulting in rhagades.[2]

Fissuring of the lips ("hacking")[1,3] and encroachment of normal skin on the vermilion border of the lips (the Wile sign)[2] may also occur. Rhagades are also seen in scleroderma and in people who habitually purse their lips over a period of years.[2] Antibiotic treatment of infantile syphilids has today made luetic rhagades quite rare.[4]

"Late" manifestations of congenital syphilis are those that appear after age 2. They may be the result of either continuing infection (*eg*, the Higouménakis sign TH-005) or the abnormal development of structures damaged by the congenital infection (*eg*, Hutchinsonian teeth MO-701, saber shins EX-602, Clutton joints EX-406).[5]

(1) Modern Clinical Syphilology. 3rd ed. JH Stokes et al (eds). Philadelphia: Saunders (1944). pp 1101-1104, 1105.
(2) Arch Dermatol. **99**: 599-610 (1969). Clinical signs of congenital lues.
(3) Labial grooving is seen in erythropoietic protoporphyria, presumably as a result of damage by the sun [The Metabolic Basis of Inherited Disease. 5th ed. JB Stanbury et al (eds). New York: McGraw-Hill (1983). p 1333].
(4) Arch Dermatol. **102**: 78-83 (1970). Clinical signs of congenital lues, again.
(5) Medical Microbiology and Infectious Diseases. A Braude. Philadelphia: Saunders (1981). p 1217.
(–) In 1986, 1 in 10,000 live-born U.S. infants had congenital lues. [MMWR. **37(S-1)**: 1-13 (1988).]

---

* *Peutz-Jeghers syndrome*[1,2]

This is one of the familial intestinal polyposes; inheritance is autosomal dominant. Polyps may occur in any part of the gastrointestinal tract, but jejunal polyps are a consistent feature. Being hamartomas, they are not themselves premalignant; intussusception and bleeding are the usual symptoms.[2] An increased risk of cancer is present, however, in the upper GI tract (stomach to mid-jejunum) and, perhaps, the ovaries.[3]

The lip spots, also found on the digits and buccal mucosa, are melanin deposits. They reside on and about the vermilion surfaces of the lips[4] and have a striking appearance: "If one looks at the lips, he might suppose that the victim had splashed through some kind of chocolate mud, wiped most of it off the face, except around the mouth and lips, leaving a stain as the only important residue.... The spots around the lip look very dark, often nearly black."[5]

Polyps occasionally occur in extraintestinal sites such as the esophagus, bronchus, nose, bladder, ureter, and renal pelvis. There may be a dissociation of signs within the same family (for example, only spots in the father, and only polyps in the son).[2]

(1) New Engl J Med. **241**: 993-1005, 1031-1036 (1949). The classic papers.
(2) McKusick 17520. Reference 5 calls it the Hutchinson-Peutz-Jeghers-McKusick-Katz syndrome.
(3) "Gastrointestinal polyps." JA Collins & CF Snow. In: Scientific American Medicine. E Rubenstein & DD Federman (eds). New York: Scientific American (6/88). 4:XIII:5.
(4) Hamilton Bailey's Demonstrations of Physical Signs in Clinical Surgery. 17th ed. A Clain (ed). Bristol, UK: Wright (1986). pp 111, 112. Illustration.
(5) Rare Diseases and Lesions. WB Bean. Springfield, IL: Thomas (1967) pp 19-20.

(Hutchinson teeth)

* *late congenital syphilis*

"Practically pathognomonic" of congenital syphilis, the shape of the entire tooth, rather than the notch alone, is characteristic. Unlike normal teeth, the Hutchinson incisor is broader at the gum than at the biting edge, giving it a "screwdriver" appearance. The tooth is shorter and narrower than normal, but is thickened in the anteroposterior dimension. The notch, when present, is half-moon shaped.[1] Traumatized teeth and those of congenital ectodermal defect may be confused with Hutchinson teeth.[2]

Only permanent teeth show changes definitely characteristic of congenital syphilis, but x-rays can be diagnostic in patients as young as 2 years old by disclosing unerupted teeth with the characteristic shape. (The developing teeth buds are damaged by spirochetes prenatally.) The upper central incisors are affected far more frequently than other teeth, but the [lower] 6-year molars may display a different malformation: four dwarfed cusps recessed within a bulging crown of enamel. These "mulberry molars" or "Moon molars" are usually early victims of decay.[1]

Hutchinsonian teeth, interstitial keratitis, and labyrinthine deafness comprise the Hutchinson triad of late congenital syphilis. Card MO-003 distinguishes early from late congenital lues.

(1) Modern Clinical Syphilology. 3rd ed. JH Stokes et al (eds). Philadelphia: Saunders (1944). pp 798-799, 1120-1127. Copiously illustrated.
(2) Arch Dermatol. **99**: 599-610 (1969). Clinical signs of congenital lues. Illustrated.

Mouth - Teeth and Gums

MO-702

Lipstick on teeth

Mouth - Teeth and Gums

MO-703

Fillings that project above the surface of the teeth

Mouth - Teeth and Gums

MO-704

Blue line on the gum,
abutting on the teeth

* *xerostomia*

Most lipsticks have hydrophobic vehicles, hence they do not ordinarily stick to the teeth. In the Sjögren syndrome, as well as other conditions that cause xerostomia (such as dehydration or use of tricyclic antidepressants), lipstick that is placed on the lips can easily stick to dry, unlubricated teeth, particularly the upper incisors.[1]

Unusual distributions of dental caries may be another effect of chronic xerostomia, due to the loss of saliva's protective effects. Ordinarily, caries are unusual in the mandibular incisor area and on the incisal surfaces of all anterior teeth, yet a woman with Sjögren syndrome was found to have extensive caries in exactly these areas. Furthermore, the major attack on the incisors apparently originated on the incisal (biting) surfaces, similar to the pattern seen in cases of congenital dysfunction of the major salivary glands. What little saliva the woman had accumulated near the molars, which were spared from the attack.[2] Many patients with the Sjögren syndrome are edentulous.

Xerostomia can slow dissolution of sublingual nitroglycerin tablets, resulting in delayed relief of angina. Chewing gum at the same time may help.[3]

(1) New Engl J Med. **315**: 1030-1031 (1986). Claims the sign appears in "most" Sjögren patients.
(2) Oral Surg Oral Med Oral Pathol. **21**: 34-38 (1966). Impressive photos.
(3) New Engl J Med. **309**: 985 only (1983). Obviously, treating the xerostomia works, too.

(perimolysis)

* *bulimia*[1,2]

The three physical signs of bulimia are (1) parotid enlargement; (2) calluses, scarring, or ulceration over the dorsum of the hand (the Russell sign), which may be commoner in the early stages of the disease, before the patient learns to vomit reflexively; and (3) dental erosion, caused by frequent passage of acid-containing vomitus over the teeth.[1]

"The erosion classically involves decalcification of the lingual, palatal, and posterior occlusal surfaces of the teeth, a pattern indicating that the acid is coming from the back of the mouth. Amalgams can be seen projecting above the surface of the teeth, because they are relatively resistant to acid, and there is absence of stain and a smooth appearance to the tooth surface."[1]

A minimum vomiting frequency of thrice weekly over 4 years will result in enamel erosion in most people. The enamel loss is irreversible. "Vigorous brushing after vomiting should be avoided because this may actually promote enamel loss." There appears to be some benefit to post-vomiting mouth rinses and to using bicarbonate rinses.[1]

(1) Ann Intern Med. **107**: 71-77 (1987). Wonderful article on the medical complications of bulimia.
(2) Am Fam Physician. **27(4)**: 199-200 (1983). Illustrations.

(Burton sign[1,2,3]) (halo saturnis[4])

* *heavy metal toxicity:*[2] *lead,*[1,2,5] *bismuth,*[2] *mercury,*[2] *gold,*[4] *silver,*[4] *thallium,*[6] *copper*[7]

The "blue line" is a series of grey-black dots about 1 mm from the free margin of the gum. It is best seen with a magnifying glass and with a corner of white paper behind the gingival border.[8] Increased capillary permeability in [inflamed] gingivae permits perivascular accumulation of metal.[2] The sign does not appear if the teeth are absent.[8]

(1) Classic Descriptions of Disease. 3rd ed. R Major. Springfield, IL: Thomas (1945). pp 324-325. Burton's 1840 description of 50 patients is reprinted in this excellent book.
(2) Differential Diagnosis of Oral Lesions. 3rd ed. NK Wood & PW Goaz. St. Louis: Mosby (1985). pp 227-228. Illustrated.
(3) Hamilton Bailey's Demonstrations of Physical Signs in Clinical Surgery. 17th ed. A Clain (ed). Bristol, UK: Wright (1986). p 118. Illustration.
(4) Difficult Diagnosis. HJ Roberts. Philadelphia: Saunders (1958). p 24 of Atlas. Illustrated.
(5) In a modern series of 31 patients with occupational lead exposure and chemical signs of lead intoxication, the lead line was seen only once [Medicine. **62**: 221-247 (1983). Excellent review of adult inorganic lead intoxication.]
(6) Cecil Textbook of Medicine. 16th ed. JB Wyngaarden & LH Smith (eds). Philadelphia: Saunders (1982). p 2225.
(7) Medical Diagnostic Signs: A Reference Collection of Eponymic Bedside Signs. RB Birrer & CD Birrer. Springfield, IL: Thomas (1982). p 21.
(8) DeGowin & DeGowin's Bedside Diagnostic Examination. 5th ed. RL DeGowin. New York: Macmillan (1987). pp 147-148.
(–) A red line rimming the teeth is said to be the Fredericq sign of pulmonary tuberculosis [Clinical Diagnostic Pearls. JC Birnholz & PE Michelson. Flushing, NY: Medical Examination (1971) p 27.].
(–) Dental crowns may cause a silver discoloration of nearby gums [JAMA. **246**: 2245 only (1981).].

Mouth - Tongue MO-801

Unusual facility in touching tongue to nose

Musculoskeleton MU-001

Stooped posture,
including flexion of hips, knees, and lower back

Musculoskeleton MU-002

Neoplasms prone to metastasize to bone

(mnemonic)

(Gorlin sign)

* *Ehlers-Danlos syndrome*

"At least 50% of patients with Ehlers-Danlos syndrome have the ability to touch the nose with the tongue, an ability manifested by about 8 to 10 percent of ostensibly normal persons."[1]

Some readers may recall that the "Candid Camera" television show did a memorable feature on this (though they did not mention the medical significance of it). They could find only one individual with the ability.

(1) Syndromes of the Head and Neck. RJ Gorlin & JJ Pindborg. New York: McGraw-Hill (1964). pp 196, 197. Illustrated.
(–) Heritable Disorders of Connective Tissue. 4th ed. VA McKusick. St Louis: Mosby (1972). p 307.
(–) Textbook of Rheumatology. 2nd ed. WN Kelley et al (eds). Philadelphia: Saunders (1985). pp 1628-1629. Illustrated.

(simian stance)

* *spinal stenosis*

The lumbar flexion afforded by the simian stance will decrease pressure on the spinal cord caused by masses at the posterior aspect of the spinal canal (typically, osteophytes). This postural adapation may prove insufficient when the patient straightens up to walk; the consequent development of neurogenic pain may be misinterpreted as the intermittent claudication of peripheral vascular disease or as disease of the hip joint(s).[1]

The minimal lumbar flexion afforded by pushing a shopping cart or lawnmower can also relieve symptoms. Of 68 patients with lumbar stenosis seen at the Mayo Clinic, 94% had this "pseudoclaudication."[2] Because humans ride bicycles and walk uphill with flexed lumbar spines, patients may have excellent tolerance for these exercises as well.[3]

Parkinsonian patients may also find it easier to bicycle (and run) than to walk.[4] Popliteal artery entrapment can make it easier to run than to walk (card EX-405).

(1) Lancet. **II**: 652-653 (1982). Simian stance.
(2) Ann Intern Med. **103**: 271-275 (1985). Review of lumbar stenosis.
(3) Lancet. **II**: 825 only (1982). Cycling.
(4) Mnemonics, Rhetorics and Poetics for Medics. RL Bloomfield & ET Chandler. Winston-Salem, NC: Harbinger Press (1982). p 187. See also: The Basal Ganglia and Posture. JP Martin. Philadelphia: Lippincott (1967). pp 23 and 92.
(–) Loss of lumbar lordosis is, of course, characteristic also of ankylosing spondylitis.

---

* *"Kinds of tumor leaping promptly to bone"*

- kidney
- ovary
- testis
- lung
- prostate
- thyroid
- breast

Mnemonics, Rhetorics and Poetics for Medics. RL Bloomfield & ET Chandler. Winston-Salem, NC: Harbinger Press (1982). pp 8-10.

Musculoskeleton MU-003

Muscular pain 5 to 10 minutes after starting exercise

Musculoskeleton MU-004

Arthralgias in a woman with breast scars

Neck NC-001

Two quick pulsations in the right carotid
for every single beat in the left

* *McArdle disease (myophosphorylase deficiency)*

At rest or with mild exercise, myocytes use plasma free-fatty-acids and oxygen in the Krebs cycle to generate high-energy phosphates such as ATP. During more intense exercise, however, less oxygen is available, so myocytes must generate ATP anaerobically, as follows:

$$\text{glycogen} \xrightarrow{\text{glycogenolysis}} \text{glucose} \xrightarrow{\text{anaerobic glycolysis}} \text{ATP}$$

In McArdle disease, glycogenolysis is impeded by deficiency of the enzyme myophosphorylase. Thus, once consumed during vigorous exercise, the myocyte's resting pool of glucose, and hence ATP, is not replenished. Further exercise results in pain, contracture, myocyte breakdown, and even visible myoglobinuria.[1]

McArdle disease can present at any age; in most instances it is autosomal recessive.[2] Because neurologic examination is usually normal, patients are often accused of malingering during athletic training. Resting levels of creatine phosphokinase (CPK) are usually elevated.

The diagnosis is tested by inflating a sphygmomanometer to above systolic blood pressure and drawing serial lactate levels from below the cuff after repeated hand contractions. The normal increase in lactate is not seen. Other disorders of glycogenolysis (such as phosphofructokinase deficiency) will manifest the same symptoms and have a flat lactate response.[3]

(1) New Engl J Med. **312**: 355-359, 370-371 (1985). Value of high-protein diet; and an editorial.
(2) Recessive is McKusick 23260. Dominant is McKusick 15346.
(3) Handbook of Clinical Neurology. **41**: 175-234 (1979). Metabolic myopathies.

---

* *postmammoplasty connective tissue disease (human adjuvant disease [HAD])*

There are several methods used for augmentation mammoplasties. The oldest is to inject paraffin or processed petroleum jelly directly into the breast, but this can lead to severe local inflammatory reactions and gross disfigurement.[1] After 1950, rubber-like envelopes filled with silicone gel were developed for implantation. Silicone, however, can "sweat" throught the envelope, and cause systemic complications[2] (see card AB-003). More recent implants feature a silastic envelope filled with saline solution.

Most of the roughly 40 reported cases of HAD are from Japan; only 8 are in the English-language literature. Few patients developed classic connective tissue diseases. Four scleroderma-like cases (characterized by the Raynaud phenomenon, skin induration, lung disease, and axillary adenopathy) developed up to 19 years after injection augmentation.[3] In one patient each, lupus, rheumatoid arthritis (RA), and mixed connective tissue disease arose within 2½ years of augmentation by silicone-filled envelopes (two of these also had the Raynaud phenomenon).[4] One woman developed seropositive RA and Sjögren syndrome 6 years after implantation of saline-filled envelopes.[5]

(1) Br Med J. **3**: 19-22, 184-185 (1968). Silicone mastitis in topless waitresses.
(2) FDA Drug Bull. **19(1)**: 2-3 (1989). Cites: Semin Arth Rheum. **47(2)**: 112-118 (1987).
(3) Arthritis Rheum. **22**: 532-537 (1979). One case was after rhinoplasty with petroleum jelly.
(4) Arthritis Rheum. **25**: 694-697 (1982). The woman with RA also had Sjögren syndrome.
(5) Br J Rheumatol. **23**: 227-229 (1984). However, seronegative RA was diagnosed 3 years before augmentation.

(Nissim sign[1])

* *aortic dissection*

Nissim considered this sign pathognomonic and attributed it to "the difference of the rate of propagation of the pulse wave through the lumen of the artery and through its dissected coats where the blood was probably partly clotted."[1] (That is, the blood flowed more slowly through the false channel.) To affect the right carotid pulse, the dissection would have to be in the ascending aorta. The strengths of the two beats in the right carotid were "almost equal."

Likewise, unilateral reduplication ("splitting") of the sound heard over the brachial artery during sphygmomanometry has once been reported. In this case, "the pulse wave was equivocally dicrotic."[2]

It is important to emphasize the transient nature of pulse abnormalities in aortic dissection.[3]

(1) Br Heart J. **8**: 203-206 (1946). Report of the sign.
(2) New Engl J Med. **250**: 670-674 (1954). Not an especially useful paper.
(3) For example, an intimal flap may suddenly move away from the arterial orifice it is occluding, or a hematoma in a false lumen that is compressing an artery can rapidly decompress if the false lumen gains access to the true lumen. [Am J Med. **60**: 625-633 (1976).]
(–) Medicine. **37**: 217-279 (1958). Excellent clinical review of 505 aortic dissections.

Neck NC-002

Thyroid nodule in a beautiful woman

Neck NC-003

Abrupt distention and quick collapse of the carotid, subclavian, temporal, brachial, or palmar arteries

Neck NC-004

Trachea dips with each pulse

(Searls sign)

** thyroid carcinoma*

H. H. Searls, at the University of California Hospital, "described a sign which may be useful in the diagnosis of thyroid carcinoma. According to Searls, the thyroid nodule in a female patient who is beautiful is likely to be carcinoma.... This sign cannot be used by older physicians since to them all women may appear to be beautiful."[1] No other information is given. Perhaps Searls is really referring to the well-known fact that nodules are more likely to be malignant in younger patients.

Curious also is this sentence by hepatologist Sheila Sherlock: "Patients with chronic active hepatitis or Wilson's disease tend to be younger [than patients with cirrhosis] and to be physically attractive."[2]

The most well-entrenched link between disease and pulchritude, however, is in the syndrome of testicular feminization, where a "very feminine phenotype" is the result of elevated estradiol levels and resistance to androgens.[3]

(1) Carcinoma of the Thyroid Gland. S Lindsay. Springfield, IL: Thomas (1960) pp 26-27.
(2) Diseases of the Liver & Biliary System. 6th ed. S Sherlock. Oxford: Blackwell (1981) p 404.
(3) Case Studies in Endocrinology for the House Officer. WM Burch. Baltimore: Williams & Wilkins (1987). pp 159-167. Testicular feminization is McKusick 31370. See also card SK-303.

(Corrigan pulse)
(water hammer pulse)

** aortic regurgitation (AR)*
** any high-output cardiac condition with large stroke volume*

This effect, due to the combination of left ventricular hypertrophy and valve leakage, was described by Corrigan in 1832.[1] It is technically incorrect to label the radial pulse as a Corrigan pulse, as he did not mention the pulses at the wrist.[2] The "water hammer" (a term introduced in 1843) was a toy consisting of a small amount of water in a wide glass tube evacuated of air. When inverted, the water struck the dependent end of the tube with "a hard, short knock, as if it were a mass of lead."[1,2]

Patients with severe AR generally wear loose-fitting collars to minimize the pounding sensations from the carotids. To avoid drawing attention to their pulsating necks, some women shun necklaces and may also dress in clothes with high necklines. Some men won't wear bow-ties because they pulsate or otherwise draw attention to their necks.[3,4]

(1) Cardiovascular Pathology. REB Hudson. Baltimore: Williams & Wilkins (1965). **1**: 1050-1054; **3**: 585-586.
(2) Clinical Heart Disease. S Oram. London: Heinemann (1971). p 358.
(3) Ann Intern Med. **47**: 27-38 (1957). Unusual manifestations of AR; antedates valve replacements.
(4) Chest. **73**: 539-542 (1978). Uncomfortable cannon "a" waves of the jugular pulse in a patient with a VVI pacemaker.

(tracheal tug)

** aneurysm or dilatation of the aortic arch*

The dilated aorta pushes down on the left mainstem bronchus, which then tugs other tracheolaryngeal structures down with it.[1,2] (Thus, aneurysms of the ascending portion of the arch do not cause tugging.[3]). "The sign is best elicited by having the patient extend the neck and close the mouth while the examiner's thumb and forefinger draw the cricothyroid cartilage upward."[2,4,5]

To be of diagnostic value, a *marked* tug must be present during both inspiration and expiration.[3] Tumors near the aortic arch are said to occasionally produce the sign.[2]

Perhaps a more specific manifestation of aortic arch aneurysm is the "tracheal diastolic shock," felt as a distinct, sharp impulse following the tracheal tug, coincident with closure of the aortic valve.[3]

(1) DeGowin & DeGowin's Bedside Diagnostic Examination. 5th ed. RL DeGowin. New York: Macmillan (1987). p 447.
(2) Medical Diagnostic Signs: A Reference Collection of Eponymic Bedside Signs. RB Birrer & CD Birrer. Springfield, IL: Thomas (1982). p 16. The Oliver sign.
(3) Am J Med Sci. **119**: 10-14 (1900). Describes the tracheal diastolic shock.
(4) However, Osler says "the patient should sit up with the head inclined forward, so as to completely relax the neck" [The Principles and Practice of Medicine. W Osler. New York: Appleton (1892). pp 673-677.].
(5) And while you have the patient's mouth closed, auscultate over his or her closed lips. The presence of a rhythmical murmur is the Sansom sign of thoracic aortic aneurysm [reference 2, p 87]. See card GU-002, too.

Neck NC-005

Anterior midline mass
that moves superiorly
when the tongue is protruded

Neck NC-006

Small palpable lymph node (2 to 3 mm diameter)
at the level of the
right 7th cervical transverse process

Neurology NE-001

Black cerebrospinal fluid

* *thyroglossal cyst*

"*The* sign of a thyroglossal cyst depends on its anatomic connection via the thyroglossal duct with the base of the tongue.... Request that the patient open his mouth. Grasp the swelling between the finger and thumb. Then instruct him to put out his tongue: to put it in and put it out again. As the tongue is fully protruded a certain amount of movement of all swellings in this region is to be expected, but in the case of a thyroglossal cyst the upward tug is unmistakable. With an adenoma of the thyroid isthmus this sign is negative but the swelling will move upwards on swallowing."[1]

(1) Hamilton Bailey's Demonstrations of Physical Signs in Clinical Surgery. 17th ed. A Clain (ed). Bristol, UK: Wright (1986). pp 165-166.
(–) A short review of thyroglossal cysts is in: Differential Diagnosis of Oral Lesions. 3rd ed. NK Wood & PW Goaz. St. Louis: Mosby (1985). pp 195-196, 199-201.

---

* *acute viral hepatitis*[1]

Twenty years ago it was said that the presence of this sign in a patient with hepatic disease "may be of considerable help in suggesting a diagnosis of acute viral hepatitis instead of mechanical obstruction."[1] Unfortunately, I have been unable to find a single other mention of this sign. Any help?

(1) "Evidence of hepatic disease that may be overlooked." WD Davis Jr. Med Clin North Am. **51**: 1003-1010 (1967). Part of a symposium on unusual manifestations of disease.
(–) In a patient with generalized lymphadenopathy, swelling of the posterior cervical nodes is diagnostic of African trypanosomiasis (Winterbottom sign). [Bedside Diagnostic Examination. 4th ed. EL DeGowin & RL DeGowin. New York: Macmillan (1981). p 224. Discussion of this sign is absent from the 5th edition, perhaps a casualty of the human immunodeficiency virus.]

---

* *primary malignant melanoma of the central nervous system*[1,2]

Although melanocytes occur in a number of areas in the central nervous system, this aggressive tumor is luckily very rare. The single reported correct preoperative diagnosis was made when the cerebrospinal fluid was found to be "coal black."[3,4] (The Froin syndrome (card NE-003) was also present in that case.)

By contrast, metastasis to the brain is very common with cutaneous malignant melanoma. Estimates of the frequency vary, the highest being 90% in a prospective autopsy study.[5]

(1) The Cerebrospinal Fluid. S Lups & AMF Haan. Amsterdam: Elsevier (1954). p 68.
(2) Cerebrospinal Fluid in Diseases of the Nervous System. RA Fishman. Philadelphia: Saunders (1980). p 173.
(3) Guthrie Clinic Bulletin. **19**: 19-27 (1953). Case report by AB King and HD Propst.
(4) Uncommon Malignant Tumors. J Antionades. New York: Masson (1982). pp 68-69.
(5) Cancer. **53**: 2550-2552 (1984). Review of CNS metastases from malignant melanoma.

Neurology NE-002

Delayed relaxation phase of deep tendon reflexes

Neurology NE-003

Cerebrospinal fluid clots in the collection tube

Neurology NE-004

Fixed, unequal pupils in a comatose patient

(Woltman sign)

* *hypothyroidism*[1,2]
* *neurosyphilis, parkinsonism, pernicious anemia,*[3] *sarcoidosis of the central nervous system,*[4] *myasthenia gravis,*[5] *schizophrenia*[5]
* *diabetes mellitus, glucose administration, sprue*[3]
* *propranolol, procainamide, reserpine, potassium administration*[4]
* *hypothermia, leg edema*[3]
* *normal puerperium, female sex, age*[4]

It is classically taught that delay in the relaxation phases of deep tendon reflexes is pathognomonic of hypothyroidism.[1,2,3] The sign is present in about 80% of hypothyroid patients and vanishes with return to euthyroidism.[1] It is most reliably elicited at the Achilles tendon with the patient kneeling on a chair.[5,6]

Epinephrine and exercise both shorten the relaxation time.[4]

(1) JAMA. **82**: 2013-2016 (1924). Woltman's original description of delay in hypothyroidism.
(2) J Clin Endocrinol. **11**: 1186-1205 (1951). Ankle jerk in myxedema.
(3) Mayo Clin Proc. **56**: 504-512 (1981). Neurologic aspects of thyroid dysfunction.
(4) Clin Pharmacol Ther. **10**: 199-206 (1969). Study of propranolol. Useful references.
(5) NY State J Med. **63**: 1148-1153 (1963). Technical considerations in measurement.
(6) Med Clin North Am. **69**: 863-880 (1985). Clinical aspects of thyroid disease. See p 865.

(Froin syndrome[1,2])

* *complete spinal block*

"The loculated fluid below the block clots when the fluid is drained. This reflects the entry of sufficient serum fibrinogen across capillary endothelial cells to allow clot formation. The protein concentration is generally greater than 1000 mg/dL. With complete block, the lower the level of a cord tumor, the higher the protein concentration and the more likely the occurrence of Froin's syndrome. Complete block at the cervical or high thoracic level ... is unlikely to result in clot formation because the protein elevations are much lower, in contrast to lesions at the lumbar level. Any lesion causing complete spinal block, such as intramedullary or extramedullary tumor, meningitis, arachnoiditis, or epidural abscess, may be responsible for Froin's syndrome."[2]

(1) "Inflammations méningees avec réaction chromatique, fibrineuse et cytologique du liquid céphalo-rachidien." G Froin. Gaz Hôp (Paris). (1903). Cited by reference 2.
(2) Cerebrospinal Fluid in Diseases of the Nervous System. RA Fishman. Philadelphia: Saunders (1980). pp 188-189.

---

* *glutethimide overdose*[1,2]

Fixed, unresponsive pupils are the hallmark of structural brain lesions. In *all* toxic or metabolic encephalopathies symmetric pupillary light reflexes are preserved until the near terminal stages *with the following exceptions*: (a) Anticholinergics and opiates may require a bright light and a magnifying glass to see the reflex, (b) hypothermia, anoxia, or severe barbiturate intoxication can fix pupils.[1,3]

A third exception is glutethimide poisoning, which "characteristically produces mid-position or moderately dilated pupils (4 to 8 mm) that are unequal and frequently fixed to light for several hours following ingestion of enough of the drug to produce profound coma. Fixed pupils in glutethimide poisoning do not necessarily signify a poor prognosis as they do under most other circumstances."[1]

One patient with glutethimide overdose had a 10 mm fixed pupil and a contralateral 5 mm sluggishly reacting pupil. Both became normal when she recovered consciousness.[2]

Transient anisocoria may occur during or after seizures; the larger pupil is usually sluggishly reactive.[4]

(1) The Diagnosis of Stupor and Coma. 3rd ed. F Plum & JB Posner. Philadelphia: FA Davis Co. (1980). pp 46-47.
(2) New Engl J Med. **285**: 806 only (1971). Case report.
(3) Cecil Textbook of Medicine. 16th ed. JB Wyngaarden & LH Smith Jr. (eds). Philadelphia: Saunders (1982). p 1919.
(4) Neurology. **16**: 837-840 (1966). Anisocoria and seizures.

Neurology NE-005

Comatose patient whose eyelids close gradually after they are released

---

Neurology NE-006

Downgoing toe on the Babinski test

Neurology NE-007

Mental clouding, syncope, or seizure during exercise

* *physiologic*

"In most patients with stupor or coma, as in sleep, the eyes are closed by tonic contraction of the orbicularis oculi muscles. (The situation changes in chronic coma when sleep-wake cycles return.) Lift the lids and release them, noting their tone. In unconscious patients the eyelids close gradually after they are released, a movement that cannot be duplicated voluntarily by a hysterical patient.[1] Absence of tone or failure to close either lid suggests facial nerve dysfunction on that side. Strong resistance to eye opening or rapid closure upon release, or both, can be voluntary, as in psychogenic unresponsiveness, or a result of reflex blepharospasm, which occurs in both structural and metabolic brain disease."[2]

Similar to this is the eyelash sign. Stroking the eyelashes will occasion movement of the lids in hysterical coma, but not in true coma.[3]

(1) Acta Neurol Scand. **45**: (Suppl. 36): 1-56 (1969). Neurological examination of the comatose patient.
(2) The Diagnosis of Stupor and Coma. 3rd ed. F Plum & JB Posner. Philadelphia: FA Davis Co. (1980). pp 46-47.
(3) Stedman's Medical Dictionary. 23rd ed. Baltimore: Williams & Wilkins (1976). pp 1284-1285. Indexed under "sign, eyelash."

---

* *meaningless unless one knows that the extensor muscle of the big toe is capable of function*

New Engl J Med. **301**: 1104-1111 (1979). CPC on amyotrophic lateral sclerosis.

---

* *McArdle disease*[1]

This is not "runner's high."

The enzyme deficiency in McArdle disease interrupts glycogenolysis (see card MU-003). Thus, during sustained exercise, anaerobic glycolysis cannot occur, and its end-product, lactic acid, does not accumulate as it normally does. (This can be documented at the bedside using the technique described on card MU-003.[2])

Lactic acid can be a major determinant of blood pH. Thus, the pathogenesis of the central nervous system effects described on the other side of this card probably rests on the alkalosis caused by an appropriate ventilatory response to exercise, without the usual compensating metabolic acidosis.[1]

(1) New Engl J Med. **312**: 355-359, 370-371 (1985). High-protein diet therapy; and an editorial.
(2) Handbook of Clinical Neurology. **41**: 175-234 (1979). Metabolic myopathies. Emphasizes that most patients with McArdle disease learn their limits and, within that framework, enjoy a nearly normal life (p 186).

Neurology - Mental State NE-501

"True! – nervous – very, very dreadfully nervous I had been and am; but why will you say that I am mad? The disease had sharpened my senses – not destroyed – not dulled them. Above all was the sense of hearing acute.... Hearken! and observe how healthily – how calmly I can tell you the whole story."

Neurology - Mental State NE-502

"New mother's tension" a few months after childbirth, followed by "postpartum blues"

Nose NO-001

Unfused cartilage at nasal tip

** adrenal cortical insufficiency*

The quotation is from the opening paragraph of Edgar Allan Poe's 1843 story, "The Tell-Tale Heart." It dramatizes two lesser-known features of untreated Addison disease (AD): psychosis and sensory enhancement.

Mental changes are frequent in Addison disease, occurring in 64% to 84% of cases. Negativism, poverty of thought, lack of initiative, and a depressive, apathetic mood are early symptoms that commonly antedate other manifestations of hypocortisolism.[1] Later, schizophrenia or manic-depressive illness may occur, "the type of psychosis [being] determined by the basic pattern of the patient's personality."[2]

Enhancement of the senses of taste (by 100-fold), olfaction (by 1000x), and hearing (by 20x) seems to be common in AD.[3] Regarding hearing, the integration of auditory input (*eg*, sound localization, loudness judgment) is impaired, and the sensory threshold for discomfort drops[3] (two characteristics perhaps apparent in Poe's villainous narrator).[4]

Corticosteroids reverse the sensory changes[3] and, less regularly, the psychosis.[5]

(1) Psychological Manifestations of General Diseases. I Hall & CW Richard. Jamaica, NY: Spectrum (1980). pp 141-142. Of course, hyponatremia and/or hypoglycemia may be contributory factors.
(2) Compr Psychiat. **4**: 90-95 (1963). Case report and review of 13 others.
(3) Prog Brain Res. **32**: 270-294 (1970). Sensory changes in hypoadrenalism.
(4) Those prompted to read Poe's tale should know: (1) the hearing enhancement is most pronounced between 1000 and 4000 Hz [ref. 3], and (2) the audible components of normal heart sounds (in situ!) are in the 60 to 100 Hz range, with high pitched murmurs at perhaps 200 Hz. [Cardiac Auscultation. 2nd ed. JS Butterworth et al. New York: Grune & Stratton (1960). pp 24-29.]. It is unclear if mania superimposed on Addisonian asthenia would furnish sufficient vigor to perform the evil acts recounted in the story.
(5) Acta Psychiat Scand. **Suppl. 255**: 203-210 (1974). Psychosis and Addisonism.

** postpartum thyroiditis*

Although a patient with thyroiditis may remain euthyroid, thyroiditis may also be manifest as thyrotoxicosis, as hypothyroidism, or as thyrotoxicosis followed by hypothyroidism. The dysthyroid changes may be transient or persistent.[1,2]

Postpartum thyroiditis is a common disorder; it was found in 5% of Japanese women studied 3 months after delivery,[1] and in 6% to 10% of postpartum Swedish women.[2] Thyroid auto-antibodies are frequently present. The postpartum rebound of the immune system, which is suppressed normally during pregnancy, is thought to be involved. Evidence of a thyrotoxic phase may be attributed wrongly to "new mother's tension," and a subsequent hypothyroid phase to postpartum depression.[3] Usually self-limited, the dysthyroid state generally does not require therapy,[3] but is likely to recur.

Of note, intravaginal application of povidone-iodine disinfectant (Betadine) can lead to systemic iodine absorption.[4,5] Iodine administration, in turn, is reported to cause three thyroidal complications: (1) hypothyroidism (via a persistent Wolff-Chaikoff effect), (2) thyrotoxicosis (the Jod-Basedow phenomenon), and, (3) very rarely, thyroiditis.[6]

(1) New Engl J Med. **306**: 849-852 (1982). Postpartum thyroiditis in Japan.
(2) Mayo Clin Proc. **60**: 836-843 (1985). Clinical review of thyroiditis.
(3) Medical Knowledge Self-Assessment Program VII. Philadelphia: American College of Physicians (1986). p 216 only.
(4) JAMA. **244**: 2628-2629 (1980). Vaginal absorption of povidone-iodine.
(5) JAMA. **246**: 39 only (1981). Diagnosing postpartum thyroiditis.
(6) Medicine. **62**: 1-20 (1983). Iodide-induced thyrotoxicosis.

** patient was breast-fed as an infant*[1]

This sign is attributed to Osler and his intimate friend, Egerton Y. Davis.[2] In babies who were breast-fed "the physical effects of breast pressure on the nose are ... evidenced ... in [that] the cartilages are kept separate and do not join; whereas in bottle-fed babies in whom there is no pressure on the tip of the nose the cartilages rapidly unite and, in the adult present to the finger in a single sharp outline, entirely different from the split bifid condition in the breast-fed child."[1]

Osler and Davis, typically ahead of their time,[1] also speculate on the possible long-term effects and sociologic correlates of this important maternal-infant interaction.

(1) Maryland Med J. **43**: 320-322 (1900). Osler's remarks at a dinner for Abraham Jacobi. Passages are reprinted in: [The Life of Sir William Osler. H Cushing. Oxford (1925). vol I, pp 525-526.] and in [New Engl J Med. **298**: 345 only (1978).].
(2) Dis Chest. **56**: 531-537 (1969). Davis' bibliography and Osler's coat-of-arms.
(–) JAMA. **180**: 826-827 (1962). Reciprocal shape determinants.
(–) A pathologically exaggerated form of the "bifid nose" has also been described. It can occur with ocular hypertelorism, as part of a frontonasal dysplasia, or as an inherited trait. See [McKusick 21040 & 10974] and [Plast Reconstruc Surg. **36**: 626-628 (1965). Illustrated].
(–) Interestingly, breast feeding appears to protect the infant from later dental malocclusion [Am J Prev Med. **3**: 227-232 (1987).].

Nose NO-002

Sneezes when sexually stimulated

Nose NO-003

Pruritus of the nostrils

Skin SK-001

Localized hirsutism

* *physiologic*

The nasal passages are lined with highly vascular tissue containing capillary sinusoids, making them anatomically similar to the erectile tissues of the penis.[1,2] Parasympathetic stimulation of either tissue bed causes vascular engorgement, manifest as mucosal swelling in the nose and as erection in the penis.[1] An exaggerated response to parasympathetic stimulation, whether a physiologic variant or due to vasomotor rhinitis,[3] can therefore lead to sneezing during sexual arousal.[1]

Thus, a 16th century youth sneezed at "the sight of a pretty girl"[4] and there was a 19th century man "who, when prompted to indulge in sexual intercourse, was immediately prior to the act seized with a fit of sneezing."[5] Sneezing may occur during or after coitus, but postcoital sneezing can also be the first sign of anaphylaxis[1] (card GU-004).

Increased sympathetic tone is associated with ejaculation and, in the nose, with vasoconstriction.[1] Thus, Schoenfeld, writer of a late 1960s "underground" medical column in Berkeley, California, notes that "several patients have reported relief from nasal congestion following sexual intercourse," and adds "no prescription is required."[6]

(1) JAMA. **260**: 401 only (1988). Brief treatment of sex and sneezing.
(2) Histology. 5th ed. AW Ham. Philadelphia: Lippincott (1965). p 748.
(3) Vasomotor rhinitis is a syndrome of imbalanced autonomic control of the nasal mucosa; parasympathetic activity is generally exaggerated (reference 1).
(4) Bull Johns Hopkins Hosp. **9**: 10-17 (1898). Discusses many naso-sexual connections.
(5) Anomalies and Curiosities of Medicine. GM Gould & WL Pyle. Philadelphia: Saunders (1896). p 511. Reprinted 1956 by the Julian Press, New York City.
(6) Dear Doctor Hip Pocrates. E Schoenfeld. New York: Grove Press (1968). pp 8-10.

(Wartenburg symptom[1])

* *brain tumor*

Pruritic nostrils are claimed to be pathognomonic for brain tumors, in particular for advanced tumors that infiltrate the base of the fourth ventricle. In a study of 77 patients with brain tumors,[2] 6 had the symptom. Typically, the pruritus was "ferocious and persistent" so that "patients could be seen scratching for hours. Even when unconscious they scratched their nostrils and, if restrained, tried to rub their noses in the pillow."[2]

It is thought that the itching is of central origin, a phenomenon that has been observed experimentally: Intracisternal injection of morphine in the cat produces "violent scratching, mainly of the ears, but sometimes of the nose and other parts of the head or neck" that lasts up to 90 minutes, and is not altered by sectioning cutaneous sensory nerves.[3] (It should, therefore, not be surprising to learn that, in humans, nasal pruritus is a side-effect of therapeutic doses of opiates[4] and is also useful in spotting surreptitious heroin abuse.[5])

Frequent nasal scratching/rubbing has been described as an early sign of meningitis.[6]

(1) Klin Wochenschr. **11**: 461-462 (1932). Original description; in German.
(2) Br J Dermatol. **92**: 675-678 (1975). Cutaneous manifestations of brain tumors.
(3) Physiol Rev. **21**: 357-381 (1941). Physiology of itching. Defines itching as "an unpleasant cutaneous sensation which provokes the desire to scratch."
(4) Goodman & Gilman's The Pharmacological Basis of Therapeutics. 6th ed. AG Gilman et al (eds). New York: Macmillan (1980). p 499.
(5) J Applefeld, RN. Johns Hopkins Hospital, June 1984.
(6) Revue Méd. **38**: 366-369 (1921). Similar to the nasal rubbing in the helminthoses; in French.
(-) The author experiences a "ferocious" nasal pruritus each time he flosses his upper teeth. It is not angina, however [New Engl J Med. **309**: 667 only (1983). Nasal pruritus as atypical angina.].

---

* *associated with localized hypervascularity and low-grade inflammation*[1]

For example:

- congenital arteriovenous fistula
- chronic osteomyelitis
- severe varicose veins and subsequent stasis ulcers
- prolonged skin irritation
- lymphedema (in the case reported, after radical groin dissection[1])

Another category of abnormalities is dependent on the site of the hirsutism, for example, a patch of hair in the lumbosacral area can be a marker for occult spinal dysraphism (developmental lesions that may place pressure or traction on the spinal cord or nerve roots).[2] Of course, localized hirsutism may be associated with dermatologic lesions as well, including, one would suspect, topical minoxidil use.

(1) New Engl J Med. **305**: 958 only (1981). Letter.
(2) JAMA. **246**: 2606-2608 (1981). Lumbosacral skin lesions as markers of occult spinal dysraphism.

Skin SK-002

Sudden appearance,
or rapid increase in size and number,
of seborrheic keratoses or freckles

Skin SK-003

Stiff joints and thickened skin
after
an episode of unusual physical exertion

Skin SK-004

Red macule or papule,
expanding to become an annular lesion up to 70 cm in diameter

(sign of Leser-Trélat)

* *internal malignancy*

Mere presence of multiple seborrheic keratoses on the skin is not sufficient to diagnose the sign, the dynamics of the lesions are more important. "Sudden" usually means a period of less than 1 year.[1]

Most patients are aware of the changes occurring. The extremities, shoulders, chest, and back are common sites of involvement. On the back, the keratoses may be arrayed in concentric arcs to yield a "splash" effect.[2] The lesions are variably pruritic.[1] Acanthosis nigricans, itself a sometime sign of internal malignancy, may develop concurrently,[3] as may florid papillomatosis (warts)[3] and multiple skin tags.[4,5]

Internal malignancy has accompanied the sign of Leser-Trélat in all 27 reported cases. Adenocarcinoma was the most common type of cancer (16 cases) and the gastrointestinal tract the most common site (10 cases). Usually, the lesions and the malignancy become evident at about the same time, but cutaneous changes can occur first (as with late-presenting cancers in the pancreas or ovary).[1] Evidence suggests that ectopic production of an epidermal growth factor is the cause of the sign.[4]

(1) Int J Dermatol. **24**: 359-361 (1985). Nice clinical review.
(2) From the photo in reference 1, the center of the arcs appears to be the scapulae.
(3) Arch Dermatol. **114**: 1803-1806 (1978). Illustrated.
(4) New Engl J Med. **317**: 1582-1587 (1987). Study of a melanoma patient.
(5) New skin tags develop in acromegaly [New Engl J Med. **301**: 1138-1142 (1979).].
(–) Semin Dermatol. **3**: 265-357 (1984). Entire issue on skin signs of internal malignancy.

---

* *eosinophilic fasciitis (EF)*[1] *(Shulman disease)*

About half of patients[2] have engaged in unusual or excessive physical exertion (such as jogging, weight lifting, cycling, badminton) in the hours or days before the onset of symptoms. Exercise is thought to exacerbate subclinical disease rather than provoke it *de novo*. The first symptoms are swelling and stiffness of the limbs, usually starting in the ankles, legs, or forearms, which spreads rapidly to involve all extremities. The trunk is variably affected. The skin assumes a puckered, dimpled look (*peau d'orange*). Most patients eventually develop flexion contractures.

Careful examination distinguishes EF from scleroderma. The digits are usually spared in EF, but are often afflicted first in scleroderma. In scleroderma the normal wrinkling of the skin is obliterated by collagenous hypertrophy, whereas it is preserved in EF. Further, the skin in EF is bound down to underlying tissues and cannot be picked up. Multisystem disease (as seen in scleroderma) is rare in EF.[1]

Peripheral blood shows eosinophilia of up to 64% and an elevated sedimentation rate. Biopsy discloses inflammation and marked hypertrophy of the fascia. Treatment with steroids is effective,[1] but the subsequent occurrence of aplastic anemia in "several" patients, and Hodgkin disease in one patient, makes close follow-up essential.[3]

(1) Johns Hopkins Med J. **148**: 81-86 (1981). Nice clinical discussion by Shulman.
(2) Johns Hopkins Med J. **151**: 203-207 (1982). Review; pediatric cases.
(3) Textbook of Rheumatology. 2nd ed. WN Kelley et al (eds.) Philadelphia: Saunders (1985) pp 1195-1196.

(erythema chronicum migrans [ECM])

* *Lyme disease*

Lyme disease is a systemic, tick-borne illness caused by a spirochete of the Borrelia class. Usually occurring in the summer, it has been reported in half of the 48 contiguous states (primarily the West, Midwest, and coastal Northeast).[1] In 40% of patients with ECM, the spirochete will be seen in 40% of skin biopsies taken.[2]

Lyme disease is clinically characterized by nonspecific constitutional symptoms (fever, headache, myalgia, arthralgia) as well as ECM.[1] Most patients (65%) have no symptoms referable to the lesion; the rest may have a burning or pruritic sensation, usually of mild degree.[2] Multiple skin lesions may occur. Some patients will develop complications weeks to months after the initial lesions: arthritic (intermittent large joint arthritis), neurologic (Bell's palsy, meningoencephalitis, peripheral neuritis), and cardiac (myocarditis, AV conduction defects).[3] Early treatment with tetracycline, penicillin, or erythromycin will shorten the duration of ECM and ablate the late complications of the disease.[1]

Other conditions with potentially similar skin lesions are: brown recluse spider bite (but has pain and central necrosis), erysipelas, drug eruption,[2] and the gyrate erythemas, including erythema multiforme.[4]

(1) Ann Intern Med. **101(3)**: I-152 (1984). Excerpt of: Morb Mort Weekly Rep. **33**: 268-270 (1984).
(2) Arch Dermatol. **120**: 1017-1021 (1984). 51 patients with the ECM of Lyme disease.
(3) Attempts to delineate Lyme disease's clinical stages, a la syphilis, are being made [Ann NY Acad Sci. **539**: 4-15, 46-55, 65-79 (1988). Entire volume is devoted to LD.]. See card GE-000, too.
(4) Semin Dermatol. **3**: 327-336 (1984). Reviews the gyrate erythemas, of which ECM is one.
(–) Mayo Clin Proc. **60**: 402-406 (1985). New Engl J Med. **319**: 1654-1662 (1988). Nice tick photos.

Skin SK-005

Inside a field of generalized depigmentation,
retention of pigmentation over superficial blood vessels

Skin SK-006

Giant reaction to insect bite

Skin SK-007

Expanding area of
hemorrhagic skin necrosis
in a warfarinized patient

** progressive systemic sclerosis (PSS)*

Three patients with this sign were seen at one hospital over 8 years. Though not explicitly stated in the article, it appears that skin overlying either arteries or veins may retain pigmentation in this manner.[1]

Vessels of the forehead, temporal areas, and limbs were most commonly affected. Two of the patients had active myositis at the time the lesions were noted; in the third, the hypopigmented areas became re-pigmented over the next 2 years.[1]

The pathogenesis of this sign may involve the abnormal temperature responses classically seen in patients with PSS (such as the Raynaud phenomenon). It is known that temperature extremes diminish melanin production by melanoma cells in vitro, and that, in normal subjects, the skin overlying blood vessels is warmer than the surrounding skin. Other factors, such as the increased oxygen tension associated with blood vessels, could also be responsible.[1]

Another pigmentary sign of PSS is a vitiligo-like depigmentation with perifollicular retention of pigment. Perhaps not coincidentally, the skin surrounding hair follicles has a richer capillary network than surrounding skin.[1]

(1) J Am Acad Dermatol. **11**: 265-268 (1984). Describes the sign.
(–) Pigmentation over veins is also seen with severe malnutrition (especially pellagra), stasis dermatitis, and distal to the site of nitrogen mustard infusion. See: (1) Vascular Spiders and Related Lesions of the Skin. WB Bean. Springfield, IL: Thomas (1958) pp 223-225 (illustrated), and (2) Rare Diseases and Lesions. WB Bean. Springfield, IL: Thomas (1967) pp 19-20.

** chronic lymphocytic leukemia (CLL)*[1,2,3]

Eight percent of CLL patients in one series were found to have severe, troublesome local reactions to insect bites. Each had had the cutaneous hyperreactions on several occasions, and all who could identify the responsible insect identified a mosquito as the offender. Although hyperreactivity usually develops within 1 to 4 years after the onset of clinically recognized disease,[1] it can occur as an early symptom of CLL.[2]

The reactions to the bites were marked by slowly developing induration, edema, erythema, and intense pruritus that peaked at 12 to 24 hours. The most severe progressed to bullae of up to 10 cm in diameter. Resolution took 2 to 14 days.[1]

Delayed hypersensitivity produces the sign. Primary sensitization to mosquitoes occurs in childhood. With continuing exposure, what begins as vigorous acute and delayed hypersensitivity reactions becomes blunted, leading to the typical adult response to a bite. Thus, the exaggerated reactions of CLL patients are similar to the reactions of children not yet desensitized by continuing exposure. The reason for this is unknown. Spontaneous development of delayed hypersensitivity in individuals past middle age is uncommon: Of 37 patients from an allergy clinic, and 54 patients with chronic myelocytic leukemia, and 45 normals, only 1 person (a "normal") gave a history of reactions to mosquito bites of over 20 mm in diameter.[1]

(1) Blood. **26**: 257-268 (1965). Unsurprisingly, intradermal testing with mosquito antigen was positive.
(2) Cancer Medicine. 2nd ed. JF Holland & E Frei. Philadelphia: Lea & Febiger (1982) p 1468.
(3) AIDS patients on zidovudine may have similar reactions [Arch Intern Med. **148**: 2296 only (1988].
(–) Patients with Fabry disease do not experience pruritus after insect bites, perhaps because of their autonomic neuropathy. [Neurology. **32**: 498-502 (1982).]

** warfarin skin necrosis*[1,2]

Warfarin skin necrosis is a serious, poorly understood disorder that typically occurs in the first few days of therapy, often in people who have previously tolerated the drug well.[2] Skin lesions begin as a patch of painful erythema that rapidly expands and necroses. The limbs and breasts are common sites of involvement, though any area may be affected. Biopsy shows fibrin thrombi within venules.[1]

In 1984 a patient with a history of warfarin skin necrosis was described who, along with several of his relatives, had levels of protein C that were about 50% of normal. Protein C is a vitamin-K–dependent coagulation factor that inhibits, rather than promotes, thrombosis. Like factor VII, its concentration falls more rapidly after the administration of warfarins than do levels of the procoagulant factors IX and X and prothrombin.[1]

Thus, a large dose of warfarin given to a protein C deficient patient may further reduce the level of protein C without immediately affecting the concentrations of factors IX and X and prothrombin. It is thought that this imbalance leads to a generalized thrombotic condition with an unexplained predeliction for the skin.[1]

Protein C deficiency is an autosomal dominant trait (McKusick 17686). However, not all heterozygotes manifest a thrombotic diathesis.

(1) Ann Intern Med. **100**: 59-60 (1984). Case report.
(2) Mayo Clin Proc. **60**: 673-674 (1985). Basic and clinical science.
(–) New Engl J Med. **311**: 1578-1549 (1984). Points to 17 other cases.
(–) New Engl J Med. **314**: 1298-1304 (1986). Review of protein C system.

Skin SK-008

Neglected, bedridden patient,
without decubitus ulcers

Skin SK-009

Pustule and erythema at the site of a sterile needle prick

Skin SK-010

Pigmented mole surrounded by a white halo

** amyotrophic lateral sclerosis (ALS)*

Charcot, the discoverer of ALS, remarked on the absence of bedsores in these patients. A century later, Japanese investigators found no bedsores in 202 ALS patients diagnosed over a 10-year period, including 36 who required hospital admission and 16 who died at home.[1]

The physiology responsible for this phenomenon is unclear. Both cutaneous[1] and vascular[2] changes have been noted in the disease, but attention has centered on cutaneous arterioles. Large, dilated vessels are normally occluded by low amounts of external pressure, while small, constricted vessels require higher pressures for occlusion.[3] Plethysmography in nine ALS patients showed monophasic waveforms typical of rigid sclerotic vessels.[2] Deranged catecholamine metabolism, possibly causing cutaneous vasoconstriction, has been noted in ALS.[4]

(1) Lancet. **I**: 862 only (1976). Cites: Neurol Med (Tokyo). **2**: 215 (1975).
(2) Lancet. **I**: 159 only (1978). Plethysmography in nine ALS patients.
(3) Lancet. **I**: 970 only (1976). Suggests central role of vasculature.
(4) Neurology. **30**: 98-101 (1980). Increased norepinephrine; decreased gamma-aminobutyric acid.

(pinprick sign) (pathergy)

** Behçet disease (BD)*

A multisystem disorder, Behçet disease was originally described as a chronic relapsing triad of oral ulceration, genital ulceration, and uveitis.[1] Hippocrates may have described a case.[2] Cutaneous vasculitis, synovitis, and meningoencephalitis are other common manifestations. The skin exhibits a nonspecific hypersensitivity to simple trauma, such as a needle stick.[1] From 24 to 48 hours after a sterile subcutaneous or intravenous needle stick, about 70% of Turkish patients with Behçet disease will develop erythema and the formation of a papule or pustule at the precise site of the puncture.[3] The frequency in British and American patients is much less.[4] Three millimeter erythema and a pustule over 2-mm in diameter represent a 4+ reaction; 20 gauge needles seem to work best. Pathergy does not usually correlate with apparent clinical activity of BD and may be intermittent.[3]

Thought secondary to increased chemotaxis,[2] pathergy has also occurred in patients with recurrent aphthous stomatitis and with idiopathic erythema nodosum.[5,6]

(1) Textbook of Rheumatology. WN Kelly et al (eds). Philadelphia: Saunders (1985). pp 409, 1174-1178. The pronunciation is BAY-chet.
(2) Int J Dermatol. **23**: 25-32 (1984). Review of BD.
(3) International Congress and Symposium Series. **103**: 169-172 (1986). The skin pathergy test.
(4) Ann Rheum Dis. **43**: 74-75 (1984). Pathergy in Britons and Turks.
(5) Acta Derm Venereol (Stockholm). **59**: 77-79 (1979). Pathergy in BD and in controls.
(6) And maybe in Hitler, too. [The Impact of Illness on World Leaders. BE Park. Philadelphia: University of Pennsylvania Press (1986). p 159.] See also card GE-008.

(leukoderma acquisitum centrifugum)

** halo nevus*
** malignant melanoma*

When nevus cells or malignant melanocytes come under immunologic attack, a halo lesion may form.[1] The halo, which is simply a depigmented area, probably forms on an auto-immune basis[2] (most likely, when there is antigenic overlap between normal epidermal melanocytes and the central lesion that is under attack). Normally the halo surrounds the lesion under primary immunologic attack, but not always.[1]

True halo nevi, defined as a central nevus cell nevus surrounded by a depigmented halo, typically occur in the young, and are benign. However, whenever a halo lesion is seen, malignant melanoma must be excluded. This may be difficult because: (1) A true halo nevus may form as a consequence of a distant, or even internal, melanoma; and (2) the original melanoma may involute entirely in the wake of a successful immunologic attack. Thus, patients with halo lesions (especially those past adolescence) need careful scrutiny of the central lesion as well as a complete, detailed skin examination.[1]

Hair follicles within a halo may be affected as well: A patch of white hair over a scalp nodule is a sign of melanoma.[3] The appearance of multiple hypopigmented patches after smallpox vaccination (a form of immune stimulation) is also a sign of melanoma.[3]

(1) Vitiligo and Other Hypomelanoses of Hair and Skin. J-P Ortonne et al. New York: Plenum (1983). pp 567-611. The relationship of halo lesions to vitiligo is uncertain.
(2) "Benign Cutaneous Tumors." EA Abel & EM Farber. In: Scientific American Medicine. E Rubenstein & DD Federman (eds). New York: Scientific American (4/87). 2:XI:9. Illustrated.
(3) J Dermatol Surg Oncol. **3**: 78-80 (1977). Leukoderma and malignant melanoma.

Skin - Hair SK-301

Increased frequency of visits to beauty parlors
or
hair won't hold its set

Skin - Hair SK-302

Full head of hair in a man

Skin - Hair SK-303

Healthy young woman with absent or scant axillary and pubic hair

* *hyperthyroidism*

These are (or perhaps, were) typical ways in which women manifest the development of the fine hair that is characteristic of hyperthyroidism.

MB Stevens, MD. Johns Hopkins Hospital. May 1982.

(Tom Wolfe sign[1])

* *chronic alcohol abuse*

"This [wino] is one of those stone winos whose face is so weather-beaten it looks like a pebble-grain full-brogue oxblood shoe. He has white hair, but a full head of white hair, so thick it looks like every hair he ever had in his head was nailed in for good. All that boozing and drinking ... must do righteous things for the hair, because there are no old men in the world who have hair like the winos."[1]

Tom Wolfe is a contemporary American nonfiction writer whose work is littered with surprisingly accurate medical phrases and insights.[2] In my experience, the heretofore unpublished Tom Wolfe sign[3] is most specific in men who have no frontoparietal hair recession at all. Ninety-six percent of white men experience some hairline recession within a decade after puberty.[4] Perhaps this androgen-dependent process is inhibited when ethanol's "righteous" estrogenizing properties[5] are chronically applied beginning soon after adolescence.

(1) Radical Chic and Mau-Mauing the Flak Catchers. T Wolfe. New York: Bantam (1971). p 165.
(2) For example, pp 79-108 of The Right Stuff [New York: Farrar Straus Giroux (1979)] describe medical tortures inflicted upon the Project Mercury astronauts. Can anyone confirm or deny the rumor that John Glenn had a three-beat run of ventricular tachycardia on the launch pad?
(3) In 1956 a Manhattan bus driver noted: "I have yet to see a bald-headed bum... most of the loafers have plenty of hair." (Ann Landers, 19 July 1986, Peninsula Times-Tribune).
(4) Ann NY Acad Sci. **53**: 708-728 (1951). Patterned hair loss in men.
(5) Goodman & Gilman's The Pharmacological Basis of Therapeutics. 6th ed. AG Gilman et al (eds). New York: Macmillan (1980). p 381.
(–) I am at a complete loss to explain President Reagan's hairline.

---

* *syndrome of testicular feminization*

There are three major types of human hair: (1) Nonsexual hair; *eg*, the eyebrows, eyelashes, and lower scalp hair, plus the fine hair of the trunk, forearms, and lower legs; (2) ambisexual hair that appears in both sexes at puberty; *eg*, in the axillae and lower pubic triangle; and (3) male sexual hair that appears at puberty in males; *eg*, on the face, chest, and upper pubic triangle. Growth and differentiation of nonsexual hair occurs under the influence of growth hormone, while ambisexual and male sexual hair are controlled by low and by high levels of circulating androgens, respectively.[1]

Patients with the complete form of testicular feminization are genetic males with testosterone-secreting testes. Due to a missing cytosolic receptor for testosterone, however, their cells cannot respond to the normal or supranormal levels of testosterone the testes produce.[2] Thus, both ambisexual and male sexual hair do not properly develop. Although these patients lack ovaries and other Müllerian duct derivatives, they appear to be phenotypically normal females (card NC-002); their estrogen is supplied by catabolism of testosterone and by augmented testicular estradiol synthesis.[3]

Diagnosis is important because the [abdominal or inguinal] testes are prone to malignancy. Patients may present with an inguinal mass suspected of being a hernia, or with primary amenorrhea. Cyclical estrogen replacement should follow testicular removal.[3]

(1) Postgrad Med. **77(8)**: 81-86, 90-93 (1985). Pathophysiological and clinical aspects of hirsutism.
(2) McKusick 31370. Hopefully, the term "hairless pseudofemale" is no longer used.
(3) Case Studies in Endocrinology for the House Officer. WM Burch. Baltimore: Williams & Wilkins (1987). pp 159-167.
(–) Axillary and pubic hair may vanish in hypopituitarism.

Skin - Nails SK-601

Brittle yellow nails and leg edema

Skin - Nails SK-602

Acquired peri-ungual pigmentation

Thorax TH-001

Butterfly-shaped area of hypopigmentation on the back

** yellow nail syndrome*

The yellow nail syndrome consists of the triad of deformed yellow nails, lymphedema, and pleural effusion.[1] Lymphatic hypoplasia is thought responsible.[1,2] The syndrome's three components may become manifest at widely separated times, as in the woman who developed lymphedema in childhood, nail changes in her 70s, and pleural effusion in her 80s. Through 1980, only 14 of the reported 51 cases had all three parts of the triad.[1]

Cessation or near-cessation of growth is the first nail change that patients notice. Some months later, a yellow or greenish hue comes over the nails, usually involving the entire plate. Both fingernails and toenails are affected. The nails may also be thick, smooth, excessively curved from side to side, undergo onycholysis, or show a distinct hump. Edema of the fingertips can occur as well.[3]

A variety of sino-pulmonary conditions (such as bronchiectasis, broncho-pneumonia, sinusitis) and systemic diseases (such as rheumatoid arthritis, hypothyroidism, and, most important, malignancy) have been associated with the syndrome.[4] Although spontaneous remissions do occur, treatment of the nail changes is usually unrewarding; vitamin E has sometimes helped.[3]

(1) Pleural Diseases. RW Light. Philadelphia: Lea & Febiger (1983). p 181 only.
(2) The nosology of yellow nail syndrome is unclear because of the many types of primary lymphedema (McKusick 15280-15340); yellow nails and pleural effusion have been described with all of them [Pleural Effusion. AO Vladutiu. Mt. Kisco, NY: Futura (1986). pp 287-289.].
(3) The Nails in Disease. PD Samman & DA Fenton. London: William Heinemann (1986). pp 116-118. The nails in this syndrome are sometimes known as Samman and White nails.
(4) Chest. **90**: 766-767 (1986). Illustrated case report.

(Hutchinson sign)

** subungual malignant melanoma*[1]

Subungual malignant melanomas account for 2% to 3% of malignant melanomas in whites, but for 15% to 20% in blacks. They often begin as brown to black discolorations in the nail bed, then become bands or streaks of pigmentation. Unfortunately, this primary lesion is invariably mistaken for a benign condition (such as bacterial or fungal infection, hematoma, or vascular tumor).[2] "It is generally attributed in the first instance to injury, and its diagnosis is always missed in the early stages.... It is, however, from the beginning, malignant. Careful observation will find at the edge of the inflamed nail a little border of coal-black colour, and this, however slightly marked, must be allowed to make the diagnosis."[1]

Even in the absence of the "almost pathognomonic" Hutchinson sign,[2] any pigmented subungual lesion is cause for concern. "All such lesions should be considered malignant" until biopsy proves otherwise. Most vexing is the confusion between subungual melanoma and hematoma; "many patients" swear they injured the nail bed, and some with hematoma recall no injury. A "hematoma" that does not migrate distally as the nail grows is not a hematoma;[3] 20% of subungual melanomas are amelanotic.[2]

(1) Br Med J. **I**: 491 only (1886). Original description.
(2) J Dermatol Surg Oncol. **3**: 75-77 (1977). Includes color illustration.
(3) Surg Gynecol Obstet. **124**: 571-582 (1967). 72 cases of subungual melanoma.
(–) Peri-ungual pigmentation occurs in Addison disease. [The Hand as a Mirror of Systemic Disease. TJ Berry. Philadlephia: FA Davis (1963). p 10.]

(butterfly sign)

** pruritus and scratching in all other skin areas*

In this condition, the skin changes actually have occurred on the nonbutterfly areas of the skin, which have become *hyperpigmented* as a result of the irritation caused by scratching. The "butterfly" on the back represents the area where it is difficult to reach and scratch.

This emphasizes the importance of skin irritation in the development of the generalized skin darkening sometimes seen in patients with chronic jaundice and pruritus. The butterfly sign has been reported most often in patients with primary biliary cirrhosis, as well as with scleroderma, the CREST syndrome, sclerosing cholangitis, and carcinoma of the bile duct.

Ann Intern Med. **78**: 545-546 (1973). Color illustration.
Arch Dermatol. **119**: 183-184 (1983). Illustration.

Thorax TH-002

Rosette of burns on the upper anterior chest wall, in the distribution of a collar

---

Thorax TH-003

Nontender fatty mass in suprasternal notch

Thorax TH-004

Interscapular bruit

* *narcotic usage*

This sign has an elegant pathogenesis: The user, with a cigarette in his mouth, becomes somnolent from the narcotic. The cigarette droops onto his skin, but the analgesic effect of the narcotic blocks any reflex movement. The prolonged contact between skin and cigarette results in a burn up to several centimeters in length. Ten to twenty burns may comprise the rosette.[1]

The sign is also seen in persons dependent on both alcohol and barbiturates.[2]

(1) Am J Med. **45**: 555-588 (1968). The narcotic addict as a medical patient.
(2) Heroin Dependency. B Stimmel. New York: Stratton (1975). pp 120, 123. Illustrated. The burns may appear as circular areas of hyperpigmentation.

(dewlap)

* *Cushing syndrome*[1]
* *multiple symmetric lipomatosis*[2]

These benign tumors, "up to 4 by 6 cm in size, are soft, discrete, movable and nontender, and composed of fat cells and sparse connective tissue." In patients with exogenous Cushing syndrome, they are reversible when corticoid therapy is stopped. Biopsy or excision is recommended only if a change suggesting malignancy occurs[1] (such as fixation, firmness, or pain).

The name is derived from the hanging fold of skin at the base of the bovine neck, known as a dewlap.[1]

In a series of patients with multiple symmetric lipomatosis (Madelung disease), 84% had lipomatous involvement of the suprasternal notch. Only the neck, at 100%, was affected more often. The physical consistency of the growths was not commented on.[2]

(1) New Engl J Med. **275**: 834-835 (1966). Brief clinical description of dewlaps.
(2) Medicine. **63**: 56-64 (1984). 19 patients with the syndrome, which is McKusick 15180.

---

* *acute pulmonary hypertension*[1]
* *cardiac septal rupture, congenital ventricular septal defect*[2]
* *aortic coarctation,*[3] *Takayasu arteritis*[4]
* *aortic dissection*[5]

An interscapular bruit is sometimes heard with the onset of pulmonary hypertension after a pulmonary embolism.[1]

With cardiac septal defects, the sound is described as a systolic murmur heard between the spine and the inner border of the left scapula.[2]

The murmur of aortic coarctation is usually heard "much better" over the thoracic spine than the anterior chest, because the site of the constriction (most commonly, just distal to the origin of the left subclavian artery) is remote from the precordium.[3] In both aortic coarctation[6] and Takayasu arteritis,[7] the intercostal arteries may be palpable in the posterior thorax.

(1) Bedside Diagnostic Examination. 4th ed. EL DeGowin & RL DeGowin. New York: Macmillan (1981). p 246. This is not mentioned, however, in the fifth edition (p 244).
(2) New Engl J Med. **307**: 1086 only (1982). Letter.
(3) DeGowin & DeGowin's Bedside Diagnostic Examination. 5th ed. RL DeGowin. New York: Macmillan (1987). p 385.
(4) Annales d'Oculistique. **177**: 161-178 (1940-1941). Case report and ocular review; in French.
(5) Dissections may also result in pulsatile interscapular masses. [Am Heart J. **13**: 426-430 (1937).]
(6) Bedside Cardiology. 3rd ed. J Constant. Boston: Little, Brown (1985) p 140. Visible, too.
(7) Acta Med Scand. **149**: 161-178 (1954). Refers to three cases of palpable arteries.
(–) Of course, any sufficiently loud cardiac sound may be audible between the scapulae (card HE-301)

Thorax TH-005

Unilateral thickening
of the
inner third of the clavicle

Thorax TH-006

Letter tattooed in the armpit

Thorax TH-007

Shoulder pain after a few minutes (say, 10)
in Trendelenburg position

(Higouménakis sign)

* *late congenital syphilis*[1,2]

* *rickets*[1]
* *clavicular fracture due to birth trauma, with later healing and thickening*

The thickening is a result of syphilitic osteitis.

Because the inner third of the clavicle arises from a nucleus that appears between the 18th and 20th years, it is hypothesized that the occurrence of the sign indicates activity of the congenital infection in adult life. (Card MO-003 distinguishes "early" and "late" congenital syphilis.) Thus, the sign should not be present in patients adequately treated in infancy or childhood.[3]

The frequency of the sign in cases of late congenital syphilis has been quoted at values ranging from 4% to 100%.[1,2,3] The thickening tends to be on the right side in right-handed persons, and on the left in southpaws.[1,3]

(1) Arch Dermatol. **102**: 78-83 (1970). Clinical signs of congenital lues.
(2) Arch Dermatol. **99**: 599-610 (1969). Ditto. Illustrated.
(3) Modern Clinical Syphilology. 3rd ed. JH Stokes et al (eds). Philadelphia: Saunders (1944). pp 795, 1083, 1130-1131. Illustrated.

---

* *patient was in the German S.S. in World War II*

Tattooing was forbidden in Nazi Germany. "The *corps d'élite*, however, received special dispensation. Thus the S.S. were compelled to have their blood-group tattooed in the axilla to assist priority in surgical contingencies. Among the Allied Forces the Russians alone were shrewd enough to realize this and they forced their German prisoners to strip and hold up their arms. Those with this tattooed identification were shot. When it became clear how the war was going, some of the S.S. anticipated this eventuality by demanding plastic surgery. In turn this merely led to the Russians taking violent action when an axillary scar was discovered, without further enquiry."[1]

Hidranitis suppurativa can cause axillary scarring.[2]

(1) The Divine Banquet of the Braine and Other Essays. M Critchley. New York: Raven (1979). p 143.
(2) Dermatology. 2nd ed. SL Moschella & HJ Hurley (eds). Philadelphia: Saunders (1985). pp 1336-1340.
(–) For a "dictionary" to help interpret the meaning of contemporary tattoos, see: The Whole Emergency Medicine Catalog. MS Jastremski et al. Philadelphia: Saunders (1985). pp 20-21.].

(Kehr sign)

* *free liquid blood in abdomen*

The pain is referred to the shoulder from the diaphragm, against which the blood has gravitated. "Frequently the patient complains of pain in one or other shoulder – usually the left."[1] Referred pain is distinguished from that due to shoulder injury by the fact that referred pain is not worsened by movement of the joint nor by pressure over the site.[1]

This sign is most useful in determining whether the spleen has ruptured after blunt abdominal trauma.[2] Estimates of its prevalence in splenic rupture range from 7.5%[3] to 90%.[4] As little as 150 mL of free blood can be symptomatic.[4]

Variations of the sign have been noted. Pain may move from the uppermost shoulder to the shoulder on which the patient is recumbent (Galloway sign),[2] or cutaneous hyperesthesia of the shoulder may be present instead of pain (Saegessen sign).[2,5] The signs of Ballance and Danforth also pertain to intra-abdominal free liquid blood.[6]

(1) Hamilton Bailey's Demonstrations of Physical Signs in Clinical Surgery. 17th ed. A Clain (ed). Bristol, UK: Wright (1986). p 332.
(2) Irish J Med Sci (6th series): 725-735 (1946). Can also detect ruptured ectopic pregnancies.
(3) Surg Clin North Am. **43**: 445-455 (1963). 50 cases of splenic rupture.
(4) New Engl J Med. **274**: 1019 only (1966). A less-than-rigorous study of 10 splenic ruptures.
(5) Zentralbl Chir. **65**: 2179-2180 (1938). "Pressure between the sternocleidomastoid and scalenus anticus give[s] violent pain."
(6) Medical Diagnostic Signs: A Reference Collection of Eponymic Bedside Signs. RB Birrer & CD Birrer. Springfield, IL: Thomas (1982). pp 6, 24. See also "sign" in Stedman's Medical Dictionary, and cards AB-002 and AB-006.

Thorax TH-008

Paraspinal mass in a patient with long-standing anemia

Thorax TH-009

Pulsatile sternoclavicular joint

Thorax TH-010

Shortness of breath and chest pain
within the first 48 hours of menstrual flow

* *extruded and encapsulated bone marrow*

These sites of extramedullary hematopoiesis are seen in congenital hemolytic anemias such as hereditary spherocytosis and thalassemia.[1] No instances related to acquired anemias have been reported.[2]

Beck states: "Tumor-like erythropoietic masses may appear outside of the marrow cavity, often adjacent to the spine. The masses are smooth, rounded or lobulated, often multiple, and when seen in chest films may resemble large encapsulated neoplasms. At autopsy, it is usually possible to demonstrate a connection, often by narrow stalks, to the marrow of the vertebral bodies. Thus, they represent extrusion from the marrow cavity through thinned out bony cortex."[1] Other authors, however, note that autopsies may not show any continuity between bone and the paravertebral masses, raising the possibilities that (1) a previously existing continuity became obliterated, or (2) extramedullary hematopoiesis arises from heterotopic or multipotential cells.[3]

About 7% of hospitalized sickle-cell patients have such paravertebral masses visible on chest x-ray.[3] Rarely, primary bone disease (for example, Paget disease) will allow marrow extrusion, leading to extramedullary hematopoiesis.[4]

(1) Hematology. 2nd ed. WS Beck (ed). Cambridge, MA: MIT Press (1977). p 238. Or see: Hematology. 4th ed. WS Beck (ed). Cambridge, MA: MIT Press (1985). p 186.
(2) J Thorac Cardiovasc Surg. **89**: 580-584 (1985). Case simulating anterior mediastinal tumor.
(3) AJR: Am J Roentgenol. **149**: 889-893 (1987). Study of sickle-cell anemia.
(4) New Engl J Med. **304**: 1411-1421 (1981). A CPC on extramedullary hematopoiesis.
(–) Medical Masqueraders. E Ask-Upmark. Stockholm: Scandinavian Univ. Books (1969). pp 82-83. Illus.

---

* *aortic dissection*[1]

* *persistent right aortic arch*[2]
* *rupture of saccular aneurysm of the aortic arch*[2]
* *aneurysm of innominate, carotid, or subclavian artery*[2]

This sign, which may occur on either side, is useful only when present.[1] In a series of 53 dissections of the proximal aorta, the sign was noted once, and not at all in 71 patients with distal dissection.[3]

(1) J Am Med Assn. **148**: 1209-1212 (1952). Describes the sign.
(2) DeGowin & DeGowin's Bedside Diagnostic Examination. 5th ed. RL DeGowin. New York: Macmillan (1987). p 246.
(3) Am J Med. **60**: 625-633 (1976). 124 patients with dissection.
(–) Pulsations in the supraclavicular fossa or the suprasternal notch may occur as a result of aortic dissection [Medicine. **37**: 217-279 (1958). p 254.]. One man had a pulsatile manubrial mass at age 23 and again at age 56. They were not aneurysms, but a cyst and a thymoma, respectively [Lancet. **II**: 287-289 (1956).]. See also card GE-003.

---

* *catamenial pneumothorax*

Forty cases of pneumothorax associated with menstruation had been reported through 1980. The initial pneumothorax usually does not occur until after age 30; only 5% are before age 25. Respiratory symptoms classically develop 24 to 48 hours after the onset of menstrual flow. The pneumothoraces are usually recurrent (unless ovulation is suppressed) and right sided (though left sided and bilateral cases occur).[1,2]

The pathogenesis is uncertain. One theory is that pleural implants of endometrial tissue cause minute pleural rupture.[1] Another believes that ectopic endometrial tissue in the thorax swells in response to ovarian steroids and impinges on a nearby bronchiole to create a one-way valve, which in turn causes localized hyperinflation and eventual rupture.[2] A third hypothesis implicates air entering the peritoneal cavity by way of the genital tract, then passing through a diaphragmatic defect into the thorax.[1] In support of this, men with pneumoperitoneum have been known to have right-sided pneumothorax.[3]

(1) Chest. **77**: 107-109; **78**: 480-482 (1980). Case reports.
(2) Obstet Gynecol. **50**: 223-231 (1977). Case reports.
(3) Br J Tuberculosis. **46**: 30-36 (1952). Cited by reference 1.
(–) Pleural Diseases. RW Light. Philadelphia: Lea & Febiger (1983) pp 195-196.
(–) New Engl J Med. **318**: 1601-1610 (1988). CPC on the differential diagnosis of pneumothorax.

Thorax TH-011

Axillary freckling

Thorax - Breast TH-201

Appearance of multiple small raised papules in the areola

Thorax - Breast TH-202

[Unilateral] gynecomastia in an older man

(Crowe sign[1])

* *neurofibromatosis 1 (NF1)*[2]

A cardinal sign of NF1, the freckles appear as a cluster or clusters of small (1 to 3 mm) hyperpigmented macules similar in color to café-au-lait spots (CLS). They are thought to be pathogenically different from CLS.[3]

Two patterns of freckling are seen in NF1: (1) Diffuse involvement of the trunk and proximal extremities, and (2) predominance in intertriginous areas (axillae, perineum, upper eyelids, inframammary region, and abdominal skin folds). Areas chronically constricted by clothes, such as the base of the neck where collars rub, may also be freckled.[3] Two thirds of the NF1 patients followed at Baylor have these freckles,[3] which are seen only when other evidence of hyperpigmentation (CLS or melanoderma) is present.[1] (The cutaneous manifestations of NF are far more varied and subtle than the simple, but well-known, rule about five café-au-lait spots.[1,4])

(1) Ann Intern Med. **61**: 1142-1143 (1964). Axillary freckling in NF. Original description.
(2) Card FA-003 distinguishes NF1 (McKusick 16220) from NF2 (McKusick 10100).
(3) Neurofibromatosis. VM Riccardi & JE Eichner. Baltimore: Johns Hopkins (1986). pp 56-75, 187, 242. Excellent book from the NF program at Baylor.
(4) Ann NY Acad Sci. **486**: 45-56 (1986). Revises café-au-lait spot criteria for NF.
(–) Arch Dis Child. **42**: 303-310 (1967). Axillary freckles in Watson syndrome.
(–) The freckle-like axillary pigmentation seen in Dowling-Degos disease may become more pronounced after emotional stress, at least early in the disease. [J Cutan Path. **7**: 77-87 (1980).]
(–) The famous "Elephant Man" probably had the Proteus syndrome (McKusick 17692), not NF [Science News. **132**: 55 only (1987).].

(Montgomery follicles)

* *pregnancy*

Also described as "large goose-pimples,"[1] this useful early sign of pregancy (especially in the primigravida)[2] is caused by hypertrophied sebaceous glands, which, more often than not, surround the orifice of an apocrine gland.[1,3] The tubercles lie at the periphery of the areola or outside it, depending on the individual.[1]

In ancient Mesopotamia (3000-6000 BC), the number of openings on the nipple of an expectant mother had prognostic significance: 5 to 6 were bad, 7 to 10 were good[4] ("thelomancy"). Modern anatomists, however, state there are "only between five and seven openings on the nipple surface that lead from the breast parenchyma" and that they are slit-like and lack pain receptors. Other orifices, of unspecified number, are round and contain pain receptors, and are the openings of sebaceous glands.[1]

Other early signs of pregnancy include: (1) Dilatation of the superficial veins of the breast,[5] (2) pulsation of the lateral fornices,[5] (3) softening of the lower uterine segment (Hegar sign),[2] and (4) bluish discoloration of the cervix or vagina (Chadwick sign).[2]

(1) The Apocrine Glands and the Breast. MBL Craigmyle. Chichester, UK: Wiley (1984). pp 57-71.
(2) Obstetrics. 2nd ed. KR Niswander. Boston: Little-Brown (1981). pp 43-48.
(3) Mosby's Guide to the Physical Examination. HM Seidel et al. St. Louis: Mosby (1987). pp 347, 356. Illustrated.
(4) The Healing Hand. G Majno. Cambridge, MA: Harvard (1975). pp 36-37.
(5) Br Med J. **1**: 593-595 (1971). One paragraph on early signs & symptoms of pregnancy.
(–) Montgomery follicles also appear on nonpregnant patients with "odontoonychodysplasia with alopecia." [Ectodermal Dysplasia: A Clinical Genetic Study. N Freire-Maia & M Pinheiro. New York: Alan R. Liss (1984). pp 95-97.]

---

* *sex partner uses estrogen-containing vaginal cream*[1]

Ten months after a previously healthy 70-year-old man's left breast was removed because of an unexplained mass, the right breast began enlarging. The cause remained undetermined after extensive evaluation. The patient was then "struck" with the fact that his wife, long a user of a 0.01% dienestrol vaginal cream for atrophic vaginitis, had in the past year routinely started to use the cream as a lubricant to facilitate intercourse two to three times a week. The estrogen exposure was stopped, and 3 months later the gynecomastia was gone.[1,2] Estrogens are cutaneously well absorbed,[3] but the dose administered via the penis in this case is unknown.[1]

Other mechanisms of venereal drug transfer exist; for example, topical medications used to treat vaginitis can cause contact dermatitis of a sex partner's penis.[4] (See card GU-004 as well.) Sex need not occur: An infant with unexplained somnolence after sleeping with his hypertensive parents was found at bath time to have a wayward clonidine patch stuck to his back.[5]

Finally, a man rubbed one of his transdermal nitroglycerin patches on his penis and produced an erection. He then had intercourse with his wife, who, several minutes later, developed "the worst headache of her life."[6]

(1) New Engl J Med. **302**: 1089-1090 (1980). Case report.
(2) Lancet. **I**: 468 only (1988). Similar cases, involving the partner's systemic use of estrogens.
(3) Goodman & Gilman's The Pharmacological Basis of Therapeutics. 6th ed. AG Gilman et al (eds). New York: Macmillan (1980), p 1427. The dose would depend, in part, on the surface area involved. Gynecomastia has also occured in ungloved factory workers handling diethylstilbesterol.
(4) JAMA. **245**: 2532 only (1981). Case report. (5) New Engl J Med. **314**: 1120-1121 (1986). Letter.
(6) Ann Intern Med. **103**: 804 only (1985). Case report.

Vital Signs VI-001

High fever and slow pulse

Vital Signs VI-002

Patient in shock
with
bullous skin lesions

Vital Signs - Temperature VI-701

Acute febrile illness
with
headache and myalgia

(temperature-pulse dissociation) (relative bradycardia)

* *drug fever,*[1,2] *typhoid fever,*[1] *yellow fever*[1,3]

* *other infectious*[4] *and non-infectious*[5] *conditions*

Practical application of this sign is complicated by two major considerations:

1. *The relative prevalences of diseases.* With typhoid fever and yellow fever now rare in temperate zones, drug fever is today the most common of the many causes for temperature-pulse dissociation.[1]

2. *The physiologically inconstant relationship between temperature and pulse.* One source[6] states that the pulse (P) rises by 8/min for each degree C, while another[1] says, for temperature (T) $\geq$ 38.9°C: $P = 15 \times (T - 38.9) + 130$.[7] Disorders of the sino-atrial or atrioventricular nodes, use of conduction-slowing drugs (for example, β-blockers), or consumption of cigarettes or hot drinks[8] can upset the "normal" temperature-pulse relationship.

(1) Heart & Lung. **13**: 460-465 (1984). Essay on selected aspects of fever.
(2) Postgrad Med. **80(5)**: 123-129 (1986). Drug fever; also notes how well drug fever patients look.
(3) Yellow Fever. GK Strode (ed). New York: McGraw-Hill (1951). pp 390-396, 416. "Faget sign."
(4) Including: dengue, Legionairre disease, leptospirosis, Rocky Mountain spotted fever, psittacosis [ref. 1]; typhoidal tularemia [New Engl J Med. **313**: 36-42 (1985).]; and Mediterranean spotted fever [Annales Derm Venereol. **110**: 909-914 (1983).].
(5) Including: factitious fever [ref. 1], increased intracranial pressure [ref. 1], and lymphoma [ref. 2].
(6) Stedman's Medical Dictionary (1976), under "rule, Liebermeister."
(7) In degrees Fahrenheit, the equation is: For $T \geq 102$, $P = 10 \times (T-102)+130$.
(8) Ann Intern Med. **98**: 559-560 (1983). Interferes with proper measurement of oral temperature.
(–) Is it true that Osler invented the modern bedside chart, where temperature and pulse are simultaneously plotted, so that temperature-pulse dissociations would be easy to spot?

---

* Vibrio vulnificus *sepsis*[1,2]

This gram-negative rod is usually acquired by eating raw seafood containing the organism or by getting seawater in a wound or in the ears. Virtually all patients who become septic have an underlying chronic disease, especially liver disease and, more notably, hemochromatosis. Increased iron availability appears to enhance virulence: The LD_{50} is 10^6 organisms in normal mice and *1* in iron-loaded mice![1]

"One third of patients are in shock when first seen clinically or become hypotensive within 12 hours of hospital admission. Over 70% have distinctive bullous skin lesions; such lesions should strongly suggest the diagnosis in patients with an appropriate history."[1] The bullae characteristically develop after tenderness, erythema, edema, and urticarial plaques have sequentially occurred.[3] Half of septic patients die, as do 15% of patients with wound infections. The incubation period is 24 to 48 hours. Thrombocytopenia is common; leukopenia and gastrointestinal bleeding are also seen.[1]

Treatment should "probably include both tetracycline ... and an aminoglycoside."[1] The organism has been found in water, sediment, plankton, and shellfish (crabs, oysters, clams) in the Gulf of Mexico and on the Atlantic coast as far north as Cape Cod. Brackish lakes in New Mexico and Oklahoma have also spawned cases. All Vibrio species will grow on routine blood culture media.[1]

(1) New Engl J Med. **312**: 343-350 (1985). Cholera and other vibrioses in the United States.
(2) Shock & bullae may appear after barbiturate (and other) overdoses [Goldfrank's Toxicologic Emergencies. 3rd ed. L Goldfrank et al. Norwalk, CT: Appleton-Century-Crofts (1986). pp 394, 546.].
(3) Arch Intern Med. **148**: 1825-1827 (1988). Brief, but recent, review of V. vulnificus sepsis.
(–) Ann Intern Med. **109**: 261-263; 318-323 (1988). Editorial and 62-case review of V. vulnificus.

---

* *Rocky Mountain* Spotless *Fever*[1]

The characteristic rash of Rocky Mountain Spotted Fever (RMSF), which usually develops between days 2 and 6 of the illness, does not always develop in adults. Probably less than 10% of all patients never develop the rash, although as many as 86% of ultimately fatal cases will not have a rash when first seen by a physician. Without the rash, diagnosis can be extremely difficult, as the differential is so large. The usual "empiric" antibiotics (penicillins, cephalosporins, sulfonamides, and aminoglycosides) are of no value in treatment. Witholding specific therapy (tetracycline or chloramphenicol) can be fatal; untreated, the mortality of RMSF is 20%.[1]

RMSF is *not* confined to the Rocky Mountain area.[2] One quarter of patients do not give a history of tick bite.[3] The peak incidence is during the warmer months of the year (however, increasing numbers of cases have been reported in April through December). Because of the danger posed by a delay in diagnosis, reference 1 advises serious consideration of a therapeutic trial of tetracycline in any adult in an endemic area with headache, myalgias, and an acute febrile illness during these months.

(1) Arch Intern Med. **142**: 1106-1107 (1982). Four fatal cases of Rocky Mountain Spotless Fever.
(2) Nor is it confined to the countryside; four cases in the Bronx are described in: New Engl J Med. **318**: 1345-1348, 1388-1390 (1988).
(3) Medical Microbiology and Infectious Diseases. A Braude. Philadelphia: Saunders (1981). pp 1458-1464. RMSF.

Vital Signs - Temperature VI-702

Episodic hypothermia

Vital Signs - Temperature VI-703

Febrile patient,
picking at the bed covers

Vital Signs - Temperature VI-704

Fever of obscure origin in a patient
living near, or working at, an airport

(Shapiro syndrome[1])

** agenesis of the corpus callosum*

In one of the two forms of Shapiro syndrome, the hypothermic episodes last an hour or two and may occur many times in one day. Body temperature (often subnormal most of the time) is vigorously lowered by profuse sweating and cutaneous vasodilation; at the close of an episode, it may be raised by shivering. Some regard this as an autonomic epilepsy. In the other form of Shapiro syndrome, the hypothermia may last several weeks.[2]

The link with agenesis of the corpus callosum is presumably a developmental one, but has been difficult to incorporate into what is known about thermoregulation in normal individuals.[3]

Independently of the Shapiro syndrome, agenesis of the corpus callosum is often accompanied by disorders stemming from abnormal neuronal migration. The diagnosis is suggested by hypertelorism, antimongoloid ocular slant, and other midline facial defects.[4] The Marchiafava-Bignami syndrome is necrosis of the corpus callosum in chronic alcoholics.[5]

(1) Brain. **92**: 423-436 (1969). Original description.
(2) Lancet. **II**: 246-247, 449 (1973). Editorial and correspondence.
(3) JAMA. **226**: 662 only (1973). Also laments the difficulty of shaking a thermometer down to 30°.
(4) The CIBA Collection of Medical Illustrations. Vol 1: The Nervous System, part 2. FH Netter. (1986) p 7.
(5) Handbook of Clinical Neurology. **28**: 317-329 (1976). Review.
(-) Br Med J. **293**: 856 only (1986). Cites recent cases; also speculates about sudden infant death.

(see below)

** ominous prognosis; seen in delirium*

This sign, noted by Hippocrates,[1] is one of the oldest observations in clinical medicine. The legion of terms for this activity (carphologia, flocillation, crocidismus, and tilmus) suggests that it was once considered to be of some importance. Little is written of it today; however, a recent study of patients with advanced cancer found that infusion of interleukin-2 and lymphokine-activated killer cells was followed by carphologia and later by "severe behavioral problems."[2] Could this be the molecular basis of the phenomenon?

Hippocrates virtually founded the bedside method, and his 42 clinical case histories (60% of which ended fatally) were almost the only records of the kind for the next 1700 years. Galen's tales, which mention his own clever diagnoses and clever cures, were written "only to puff his own reputation." Thus, apart from a few Arabian efforts, the practice of taking clinical case histories died out until the time of the postmortems of Benivieni and Vesalius in the 15th and 16th centuries.[3]

(1) The Genuine Works of Hippocrates. F Adams (transl). Huntington, NY: Robert E. Krieger (1972). Book of Prognostics, paragraph 4.
(2) Ann Intern Med. **107**: 293-300 (1987). Neuropsychiatric effects of IL-2 and LAK cells.
(3) An Introduction to the History of Medicine. 4th ed. FH Garrison. Philadelphia: Saunders (1929) pp 94-95, 97.

** malaria*

At least six cases have been reported from Europe. It is presumed that parasite-infested Anopheles mosquitoes flew aboard an airplane parked on the ground in a malaria endemic area, then deplaned in a developed country and infected humans living or working nearby.[1]

Of note is that international airports are required to meet certain minimum sanitary conditions, including a 400-meter wide mosquito-free buffer zone around the airport.[2]

By the way, the degree of attraction a mosquito has to a (human) woman varies with the phase of the woman's menstrual cycle.[3,4]

(1) Lancet. **II**: 881-882 (1982). Jet-set mosquitoes.
(2) Aerospace Medicine Primary Course, USAF School of Aerospace Medicine, Brooks AFB, TX. 27 Feb 1985.
(3) JAMA. **191**: 193, 965 (1965). What draws the beasties to us.
(4) Proc NJ Mosquito Extermination Assoc. **50**: 250 (1963). Cited by reference 3.

Wish List WI-001

1. Brown stain on the pillow in the morning
2. Malformation of the pinna
3. Shivers after urinating
4. Visual cortex destroyed, but can still see

* *These are items I wanted to include as true cards, but for which I lacked literature references. Consider them as unsubstantiated... and as homework!*

---

1. This sign of *pulmonary hemorrhage* was presented at Grand Rounds as a manifestation of Goodpasture syndrome. The brown stain represents heme-laden macrophages.

---

2. That this is a marker for *renal malformation* seems to be relatively common knowledge, but I have failed to find it in the literature. Mozart had a congenital pinnal malformation, which he concealed under long hair; it has been suggested he had kidney disease.

---

3. This is an indication that the *room temperature is below some certain point* (sounds dubious). I *think* I read it many years ago in a book about microcomputers in medicine, which I cannot now locate. A heat loss effect also seems plausible.

---

4. This phenomenon is apparently due to a (vestigial?) *visual center in the midbrain.* Interestingly, these patients typically deny their [limited] ability to see, as opposed to patients with Anton syndrome, who typically deny their blindness.

7250738R0

Made in the USA
Lexington, KY
06 November 2010